The English System

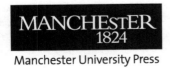
Manchester University Press

For Pedro and Mio

The English System

Quarantine, immigration and the making of a Port Sanitary zone

Krista Maglen

Manchester University Press

Manchester and New York

distributed in the United States exclusively by Palgrave Macmillan

Published by Manchester University Press
Oxford Road, Manchester M13 9NR, UK
and Room 400, 175 Fifth Avenue, New York, NY 10010, USA
www.manchesteruniversitypress.co.uk

Distributed in the United States exclusively by
Palgrave Macmillan, 175 Fifth Avenue, New York,
NY 10010, USA

Distributed in Canada exclusively by
UBC Press, University of British Columbia, 2029 West Mall,
Vancouver, BC, Canada V6T 1Z2

British Library Cataloguing-in-Publication Data
A catalogue record for this book is available from the British Library

Library of Congress Cataloging-in-Publication Data applied for

ISBN 978 0 7190 8965 7 hardback

First published 2014

The publisher has no responsibility for the persistence or accuracy of URLs for any
external or third-party internet websites referred to in this book, and does not guaran-
tee that any content on such websites is, or will remain, accurate or appropriate.

Typeset
by SPi Publisher Services, Pondicherry, India
Printed in Great Britain
by TJ International Ltd, Padstow

Contents

Tables

Acknowledgements

This book is the result of many years of work and thought on this project and others, as well as the indispensable assistance of a great many people.

I could not begin to acknowledge all those who have helped me through this process without first expressing my deep gratitude to my two supervisors at Glasgow University, Anne Crowther and Marguerite Dupree. This book sprung from my doctoral thesis, and without their constant encouragement, guidance and extraordinary patience with my younger and more impetuous self, its underlying research and ideas would never have been developed. My examiner, Michael Worboys, also gave thoughtful and lasting advice and comments. During my time at Glasgow, I was extremely fortunate to be part of both the Wellcome Unit for the History of Medicine as well as the Economic and Social History Department, and I must extend my thanks to everyone who worked there during that time. Particular thanks must be extended to Andrew Hull, Malcolm Nicolson, Ann Mulholland, Rae McBain and my fellow doctoral students, Rosemary Elliot, Matt Egan, Mark Freeman and Debbie Nicholson who provided great early feedback. Beyond Glasgow University, I received wonderful help and guidance from a number of people in the early years of this book's development. I am particularly grateful to Bernard Harris, David Feldman and Ann Hardy for their advice as I took my first tentative steps into this research. Their questions and suggestions prompted me to expand the initial approach of my research. I am indebted to Nick Evans for constantly participating in an exchange of ideas. His doctoral work on transmigration across Britain helped to fill a number of gaps in my knowledge. Patrick Wallis, Nadav Davidovitch and Alex Benchimol all pushed me to think more critically about my research and provided much needed support.

I am grateful for the help and patience of staff at the Corporation of London Records Office, the National Archives at Kew, the London Metropolitan Archives, the Jewish Museum, the Mitchell Library in Glasgow, the Wellcome Institute Library and the National Archives and Records Administration in Washington DC. Invaluable financial assistance, without which this project would not have been possible, was generously provided by the Wellcome

Trust, the Overseas Research Students Award Scheme and the Department of Economic and Social History at Glasgow University.

I am also indebted to past members of the Wellcome Unit for the History of Medicine at Oxford University where I undertook my post-doctoral research on Australian quarantine. The research and thinking I explored there and with them enabled me to build on the work that I had undertaken for the PhD. Mark Harrison, Jo Robertson, Pratik Chakrabarti, John Manton and many others in that wonderful place provided great inspiration and stimulating company in which to cultivate my ideas.

Since then I have migrated, like many in this book, across the Atlantic. Here in the United States I now find myself among a faculty of historians at Indiana University who I like and admire a great deal, all of whom provide an environment of support and encouragement. Some of them have been particularly helpful in the process of finally bringing me back to this project so that I could produce the book you now hold. They are: my marvellous mentor, and fellow Australian, Judith Allen; the brilliant Ann Carmichael; as well as Lara Kriegel, Michael Dodson, Marissa Moorman, Alex Lichtenstein, Peter Guardino, Claude Clegg, Peter Bailey and the many other colleagues who make our department such an extraordinary place.

I must also acknowledge the indispensable moral support of my friends and family who encouraged me to continue with this project when I thought I was done with it. I am fortunate that this list is long; however, it means that I can only name some of those who have cared for, encouraged, understood and put up with me. John Nieuwenhuysen has been a great academic sponsor of mine for many years and has gently urged me on many occasions to get this work finished. My dearest friends Sarah, Anne, Megan, Kai, Kat, Lucy, Garfield and here in Bloomington, Estela, Johannes and Amy, all help me to feel that the world isn't such a big place after all. Distance has been no obstacle to the love and reassurance offered by my immediate and extended family in Australia, Portugal and South Africa. Since I began this project all those years ago, my family has grown to include all the Machados, Da Silvas and Dents who are a wonderful group of people I now have the privilege of calling my own. It has also shrunk in ways that have brought and continue to bring great sadness. Four of my greatest supporters in this project and in life – Sheila Martin, Jenny Jones, and Lesley and Jack Raven – are no longer here, but I know they would be bursting with pride to see this publication. My loving parents and sister, Fay, Leo and Kobi Maglen, have maintained the essential moral, emotional and intellectual support they have always given me.

Finally I am most thankful to the two people who have been with me every step of the way – my magnificent boys, Pedro and Mio. Pedro has pushed me, reassured me, sustained me, cheered me and loved me without reserve throughout this process. He read my drafts, edited my prose, challenged my thinking and made it all feel possible. It is to him and our delightful Mio that I dedicate this book.

Introduction

Thursday, 25 August 1892, was another gloomy day. The clouds were low and heavy and the temperature had struggled to reach seventy degrees. Philip Whitcombe, Acting Port Medical Officer for Gravesend, gathered up his things and stepped into the launch. A message had just come through to his office from the Customs department that a ship had arrived from Hamburg with three cases of suspected cholera on board. This came as no surprise. Whitcombe and his colleagues had been preparing for this moment for weeks as they charted various outbreaks across Europe, appearing in one place after another. Once on board the suspect ship, the *S.S. Gemma*, it was clear that the disease had crossed the North Sea. Two women, Bessie Goldberg and the elderly Mira Janokowsky, as well as a man called Jacob Zarnobrosky were all suffering the excruciating late stages of cholera. Jacob had become so weakened by the ravages of the infection that Whitcombe feared he would not be able to survive being moved to the port's Isolation Hospital at Denton. But, with the assistance of his more senior colleague, William Collingridge, whom he had anxiously summoned along with the ambulance boat, all three were transferred to the hospital. Bessie, however, did not survive the night, and by the following evening Mira and Jacob were also dead.[1]

Having moved the three infectious cases off the ship, Whitcombe and Collingridge turned their attention to everyone else on board. After a brief inspection, those passengers who had travelled in the *Gemma's* comfortable first and second class cabins were permitted to leave, to return to the security of home or the welcome of friends, while Bessie, Mira and Jacob's forty-three fellow passengers in the cramped and dirty accommodations of steerage class, most of whom were Jewish migrants fleeing increasingly hostile conditions in Eastern Europe, were detained for a further six days of observation. The arrival of the *Gemma* tested the nerves of the two physicians as they partially implemented a new approach to public health at the ports. This novel 'English System' represented a new way of thinking about diseases which threatened to enter Britain via the ports but, they wondered, would it hold against the threat of cholera, particularly when the disease was found among poor and 'filthy' migrants like Bessie, Mira and Jacob? How and where was the boundary to be drawn against the threatened invasion? Was the disease the threat or the people who brought it?

The case of the *S.S. Gemma* marks a pivotal shift in the way imported infections were conceptualised and countered in British ports. It represents a decisive moment when disease control practices at the ports shifted away from being based on a categorisation of disease, and instead came to be based on a categorisation of person. Concepts of nation and health coalesced around the undefined space at the ports, and the heretofore under-examined connection was made in Britain between port health and the medical regulation of immigration. These are the central themes of this book.

By the late nineteenth century, Britain's ports were teeming with ships from around the world. The empire's prosperity and power were at their peak, and commercial and passenger shipping reached levels never before seen. Steam and sailing ships departed and arrived into British ports daily, loaded with goods and people from every corner of the globe. By 1892, over 10,000 vessels from 'foreign' ports arrived into London each year, with around 5,000 converging on both Liverpool and Newcastle.[2] The sea ports and harbours of the late nineteenth century were not the run-down terminals of today, where freight-ships and ferries pass by the many empty docks of Liverpool, London or Glasgow, overseen by a skeleton staff of customs and port officials. Victorian ports were swarming, busy places, where large vessels and small competed for space. Yet, amongst the cacophony of commerce and commotion, lines were drawn, hierarchies formed and diseases lurked.

Although much scholarship has been devoted to maritime history and the history of public health in Victorian Britain, there has been, surprisingly, very little written about the important link between these two subjects. It has long been acknowledged that devastating epidemics of diseases such as cholera were imported into Britain in the nineteenth century, killing large numbers of people in the most painful and degrading fashion. But most scholarly investigations which have explored imported epidemics such as these have focused on the spread and consequences they wreaked after they had taken hold within the country.[3] Public health developments in the prevention and control of infectious disease have been studied in relation to the sanitary reform and vaccination movements of the middle decades of the nineteenth century, and through the examination of medical innovations in the understanding of disease aetiology in the years that followed. The work of Medical Officers of Health has also been given increasing consideration. Yet, the policies and practices which operated to intercept the importation of infectious diseases at the ports have attracted little attention in the British context. A few scholars have contributed to the basic understanding of port health in late-nineteenth-century Britain, showing that the sanitary system of public health extended to the ports, that the health of the ports was, in the last quarter of the century, overseen by medical officers similar to those who worked in towns and cities, and that quarantine was widely detested and rarely used in the latter half of the century.[4] However, no scholarship has to date focused singularly on the transformative period of late Victorian and early Edwardian port health as a separate phenomenon within the development of public health and infectious disease prevention. Nor, importantly, has it made the crucial connection, examined in other national settings, between histories of maritime commerce and immigration and medicalised concepts of the person and State, which played out in distinctive ways in the British context.[5]

Similarly, historians of late-nineteenth-century immigration into Britain have tended to concentrate on the economic effects, responses and restrictions to immigration, paying only passing consideration to matters of health.[6] Where scholars have addressed immigrant health in Britain in this period, they have researched questions and conditions well after arrival, looking, for example, to comparative infant mortality rates, life expectancy and instances of disease in immigrant neighbourhoods and communities.[7] None of these studies has examined the medical inspection of immigrants at the time of arrival, nor how perceptions of risk, relating to immigration, affected existing practices in port prophylaxis.

In contrast to the relatively lively study of the health screening of immigrants in late-nineteenth- and early-twentieth-century America and Australia, there has been a conspicuous gap in the equivalent British history.[8] In both the United States and Australia, a number of important histories have been written about the close connection between port medicine and public health, and the policies and ideologies of immigration. Howard Markel has argued, for example, that immigration and disease control in US ports became integrated both conceptually and in practice during the nineteenth century, explaining: 'In many respects, the movement to restrict immigration to the United States during this period was a call for quarantine in its broadest sense against undesirable immigrants.'[9] British responses to the health of arriving immigrants, however, developed differently from those in the United States, which received over ten times more migrants than Britain, and from those of other places similarly studied. In each of these other examples, scholars have shown awareness that Britain forged a unique path, but its difference is mostly assumed rather than examined.

The inclusion of a clause in Britain's 1905 Aliens Act that prohibited entry to anyone who 'owing to any disease or infirmity were likely to become a charge upon the rates or otherwise a detriment to the public' at first suggests that the narrative of diseased immigrants played out in comparable ways on both sides of the Atlantic. Instead, only a relatively small portion of the vigorous debate surrounding immigration to Britain in the very last years of the nineteenth century related to the health of immigrants on arrival. Yet, it is clear from the numerous articles that appeared in *The Times*, the *British Medical Journal* (BMJ) and *The Lancet*, for instance, that there was considerable apprehension about the role of immigration in the importation of cholera and other infectious diseases. The arrival of 'Russian Jews', these publications declared in unison, 'constituted a danger to public health.'[10] Even so, these concerns were not generally echoed in parliamentary debates, nor were they central to the demands of anti-immigration political groups.

Unlike in America, the reception and transmigration across Britain of thousands of migrants in the period 1881–1905 was only answered with a call for strictly enforced medical inspections at the ports as a supplement to other concerns. The relative lack of medical rhetoric in anti-immigration campaigns, particularly when immigrants were clearly not disassociated from disease importation, suggests that something else was going on at the ports in relation to disease prevention.

What distinguished Britain in its medical response to immigration in this period then was not the origin or scale of that immigration, but its approach to port health more broadly. While immigration and port health became increasingly connected at the end of the century, the latter had developed as a separate and important focus of policy and diplomacy during the preceding decades, unrelated to immigration.

Differences in the British approach to port health and the health of arriving immigrants have not been adequately understood because the two have been assumed to be coupled in the same ways as they were in the other places examined by historians. Rather, a full appreciation of the way Britain responded to immigrants at the turn of the twentieth century requires an examination of its ideologies, systems and practices of port health more generally in the nineteenth century.

Anne Hardy showed that in the final decades of the nineteenth century a system of infectious disease prevention was established at the ports based on the sanitary system of public health. This system, which diverged from methods of disease prevention in European and American ports, established the Port Sanitary Authorities under the 1872 Public Health Act. It differed from other methods of port infectious disease control by taking the monitoring and isolation of infectious cases away from quarantine, relying instead on the sanitary condition of the ports, as well as conditions within and the cooperation of inland sanitary districts.[11]

Hardy's article remains as a staple in the still underdeveloped literature on British port health. Together with my own *Social History of Medicine* article of 2002, these two studies form the main substance of work published on the Port Sanitary Authorities.[12] They explain how the system was developed with the dual motive of preventing the introduction and spread of cholera, which had been pandemic in Europe in 1830–32, 1847–49, 1853–54, 1865–66, 1873, 1884 and 1892–93, and to provide an alternative to quarantine, which had proved incompatible with Britain's political and economic commitment to free trade. The success of the new system was, Hardy explained, 'widely admired by contemporaries' and was responsible, in addition to the general sanitary improvement of British towns, for 'holding repeated cholera attacks at bay'.[13] She argued that the success and 'professional cohesion' of the sanitary system at the ports led to 'public complacency', despite greater awareness about repeat attacks of cholera in the closing decades of the nineteenth century. This reflected a public 'confidence in the sanitary service' even though the disease remained of grave concern to medical officers.[14] By the 1880s this concern about a possible return of cholera was beginning to be linked in the medical press to the large number of migrants who passed through British ports each year, and calls were made to provide special arrangements for the arrival of migrant vessels.

The basic framework provided in this founding literature has provided an important plug in the vast hole in the history of port health in Britain.

However, we are still missing key details and, most importantly, are left with many questions unanswered and broader implications unexplored. Not least amongst these are those relating to the relationship between port health and developing concepts of nation and citizenship, as well as the links, made elsewhere, between quarantine and the drawing of national borders.

Quarantine, the most widely practised system of disease control across Europe and its colonies and the United States, had been the primary bulwark against infectious disease since the late medieval period. By the nineteenth century it had become an important tool in the demarcation of lines of sovereignty. Various states exploited quarantine's interventionism as well as its location at geographical boundaries in the process of defining national space. As the work of Alexandra Stern has shown in the American context, for example, and Bashford has asserted for Australia, quarantine was an important tool in the drawing of land and sea borders, and in the classification and identification of the desirability and undesirability of those who wished to cross those borders. Quarantine, Bashford argues, implies 'the nation' because both 'determine an internal and an external, often nominated as clean and dirty, through the administration of a boundary'.[15] The use of quarantine and medicalised lines of territoriality thus created 'geo-bodies' that sought the same protection as individual bodies in repelling potentially dangerous infections.[16] However, medicalised borders should be seen not only as exclusionary but also as inclusionary. US immigration medical examinations were, as Amy Fairchild has shown, not only intended to keep out those people who arrived with threatening illness but were also 'shaped by an industrial imperative to discipline the labouring force in accordance with industrial expectations'.[17] In such a way, medical frontiers had the dual purpose of prohibiting the entry of 'foreigners' into the national 'body' as well as regulating the admission of those deemed beneficial to it. In this standard metaphor of the embodied State the nation is ordered and contained, its boundaries sealed against infections while controlling the entrance of that which feeds it. But, just like human bodies, there are openings which act as 'points of contact and contagion'.[18] The mouth, for example, is an instrument for the intake of sustenance and for communication, but may also, while engaged in these activities, provide a means for disease to enter. If we accept this metaphor, we may consider ports as key openings into the body of the State.

As places of connection, ports were central to the application of quarantines. More than just localities for arrival and commerce, they represented sites of tension between notions and constructions of 'exterior' and 'interior' or 'foreign' and 'domestic', where the dangerous and diseased 'them' encountered the protected sphere of 'we'. As Etienne Balibar has described, a frontier 'locates a site both of enclosure and contact', and ports were the aperture where each side met.[19] This meeting place extended both outward into maritime space and inward into port towns and cities. 'If a port is more than an interface between land and water', Sarah Palmer explains, 'then a port town or city was more than just a settlement behind the waterfront'.[20] Residents of port cities interacted with the ports through business, the creation of local and civic response to the peculiarities of port and maritime populations, and through the people and goods that moved into and through them. Their character was defined by their points of contact – foreign or coastal – and the nature of their maritime activity – 'industrial and commercial' like Newcastle and Glasgow for example, naval like Plymouth or 'general cargo giant' like London or Liverpool.[21] The relationship between 'internal' and 'external' mechanisms and forces also varied depending on whether a port focused on import or export, passengers or cargo, or was a general entrepot. In each case, ports became significant 'in-between' places, where these tensions could be negotiated and where often they overlapped. Like frontiers, then, ports were and are complex constructions, being not simply the geographical or even geopolitical point of entry and exit, but places speaking to multifarious concepts of nation, identity, security and organisation.

This becomes immediately apparent when we also acknowledge that 'Britain' at the end of the nineteenth century could not simply be confined or defined by the drawing of a geographical border at the littoral. Nor would it fit neatly within the geography of the 'Four Nations' – England, Scotland, Wales and Ireland.[22] Others have suggested that 'Britain *was* the British Empire'[23] or could be more racially defined as 'Greater Britain', an aggregate of 'Anglo-Saxon' or 'British' settlements throughout the world.[24] Each of these is problematic, and it is not the intention of this book to offer any particular answer to the questions they raise. Rather, with the ports as its axis, it will show how public health responses to incoming ships and people adjusted and reconfigured understandings of Britain's borders to being more fluidly determined and shaped rather than drawn with precision at one point or another.

The model of corresponding lines of quarantine and nation set up in the Australian literature has also been problematised by John Welshman. Writing on mid-twentieth century screening of immigrants for tuberculosis, he has shown the difference in response to imported disease in Britain and its consequences for the border.[25] He argues that through the establishment of the confusingly titled 'port of arrival system' in 1965 (codified in the 1968 Commonwealth Immigration Act), immigrant screening was moved away from the ports or airports of arrival and handed over to local medical officers of health.[26] By relocating disease prevention away from points of entry and instead using medical officers to 'advise [immigrants] to register with a family doctor', Welshman argues that we cannot generalise the connection between migration, public health and the drawing of national borders. The latter, he says, 'could be moved internally – to the local level – as well as externally'. As such, perhaps it would be more fruitful to understand that 'the "border" functions more effectively at a metaphorical or symbolic level than in terms of a national frontier'.[27]

Although more than half a century beyond the scope of this book, Welshman's argument offers some useful concepts around which to begin exploring the management of port health in the late nineteenth century. However, Welshman predicates his thesis on the assumption that the idea of immigrant screening away from the ports was new to the post-war period. Consequently, the arguments he provides for the introduction of the 'port of arrival system' – that 'actual' port screening was deemed unnecessary or impractical because of the size of the problem, the anticipated costs and the possible effects that closing the borders could have on immigrant labour – remain incomplete. By extension, his argument for a 'metaphorical or symbolic' national frontier, while valuable, can be pushed further by exploring these themes in an earlier phase.

This book's examination of the pivotal period in port health, roughly from the 1870s to the first decade of the new century, offers an important antecedent to Welshman's story, pushing the fluid construction of the British geo-body back to a much earlier juncture and showing how the more equivocal border it created preceded post-war and Commonwealth immigration. A combination of port sanitation and sanitary surveillance, known to contemporaries as the 'English System', was gradually introduced as a unique alternative to quarantine. This was perfectly located in the 'in-between' space of the littoral, bringing maritime disease control within the domestic public health infrastructure, yet keeping instances of infection at a safe distance. Rather than marking a geographical perimeter, the new system identified a particularly 'English' public health zone that was more elastic and could be stretched (to include parts of the colonial diaspora) or contracted (to the coast of island Britain) to define different and changing constructions of 'national' space and those who 'belonged' within it.

But, what did 'English' mean in this context? The conflation of 'English' and 'British' certainly troubled some in this period, and there were those who worked hard to distinguish their difference.[28] However, most (in London, particularly) continued to use them interchangeably, and the use of the term 'English System' for the port sanitary system in England, Wales and Scotland clearly shows that such composite thinking still prevailed in some circles. There were variations in the administration of the Port Sanitary Authorities in England and Wales and those in Scotland were legislated and administered under separate Scottish public health laws. However, all were based on the same principles. This book explores the 'English System' within a broadly 'British' framework and approaches the history of port health in this period in such terms. Nevertheless, I recognise that variations will doubtless appear in more detailed local studies and am aware of modifications in smaller and regional ports. However, by using the 'English System' to describe the new practice of disease prevention, contemporaries sought to emphasise its divergence from the quarantines performed elsewhere and to claim that its ideals and standards were peculiarly 'English' – meaning 'British'. It therefore referred more to its difference from 'non-British' practices than recognising internal differences or seeking to define and unify something especially 'English'. Instead, it referred to an area of sanitary management which was and could be defined as singularly 'British' (called 'English'); what I call the 'sanitary zone'.

The term 'sanitary zone' has been used elsewhere within a broader literature that finds the concept of 'zones' rather than borders to be a more fruitful way of understanding national boundaries. As such, the idea of a 'sanitary zone' has been used to define an area around the border 'with mixed jurisdiction under international oversight', which was aimed at creating an 'ambivalent' or 'de-bordered' space within which refugees particularly could be processed through quarantine procedures between, rather than along, lines of sovereignty.[29] Such zones, then, are generative of a different kind of border which defies 'an absolute line of demarcation' creating a broader or more fluid space which might be conceptualised as 'a margin or zone of differentiation'.[30] This notion provides a productive framework for thinking about Britain's borders in the late nineteenth century.

Caught between the often conflicting and messy constructs of British space – the 'British' Isles, the 'Four Nations', the Empire – as well as liberal desires to facilitate the free movement of goods and people, the 'English System's' control of infectious disease at the ports did not define a blunt border. Rather, it permitted an openness to the ports that was otherwise potentially closed with quarantines, and instead generated a sanitary zone where the condition of places on either side of the littoral identified categories of inclusion and exclusion. These conditions were described as 'diseased', 'unsanitary' or 'suspected', for example, and were positioned outside the sanitary zone or made to conform within it. Disease control under the 'English System' was therefore about place – either the sanitary order of places such as urban districts, ports of departure, or on board ships; or ideas about the origin or 'natural home' of a disease.

The introduction of restrictions to immigration fundamentally challenged these underlying principles of place that had been carefully constructed in the last three decades of the nineteenth century, and that many had worked hard to establish as an alternative to the constraints of quarantine. Redirecting public health at the ports toward immigration demanded that diseases be identified and controlled not by place but within particular populations and particular bodies. This transition is a central focus of this book.

In exploring how and why these changes occurred in Britain in the late nineteenth and early twentieth centuries, the book concentrates on the Port of London, not exclusively, but primarily. There are a number of reasons for this. First of all, the 'English System' was centrally administered from London by the Local Government Board and was organised around the Port Sanitary Committee, both of which were based in the Capital. Their records, now housed at the London Metropolitan Archives, relate to England and Wales, but much of the material concerns London.[31] They are extensive and rich in detail and have not, to my knowledge, been examined in any great degree (or at all) by anyone but myself. London and Liverpool differed from all other port and riparian districts across England, Wales and Scotland in that they were the only two ports to have full-time, dedicated Port Medical Officers of Health. Every other port used the Medical Officer of Health for the port town or city as their Port Medical Officer. London therefore does not necessarily reflect the way port health was practised around the

country, but its size and the volume and nature of the shipping it serv-
iced meant that the Port Sanitary Authority there was by far the most
active. Liverpool also had a permanent Port Medical Officer, but while
a 'general cargo' hub like London, it served its industrial manufacturing
hinterland and thus, while importing raw materials, tended to be more
export than import oriented like London.[32] Therefore, as this discussion
of port health is as much about connections with spaces beyond Britain
as within, the role of London as the primary international port – the so-
called 'emporium of the world' – is central to the analysis.

In addition, but perhaps more critical to understanding the book's
general focus on London, are the particular patterns of migration to
and through Britain in the so-called 'period of mass migration' from
1880 to 1914. Unlike important Northern ports such as Hull, Newcastle
and Liverpool, London was a 'true' immigrant port, in that the majority of migrants who arrived into the metropolis remained in the city.
While immigrant communities did settle in the North and become
visible minorities, none were deemed so conspicuous or attracted as
much attention as the Eastern European Jews who settled in London.
The city received over sixty per cent of the Jewish immigrants who
arrived during these years, with most of them settling within a two-
square mile area of London's East End.[33] The Humber ports of Hull and
Grimsby, as well as Newcastle and other east coast ports, on the other
hand, were transmigrant ports. Migrants tended not to settle in those
cities in such great numbers and instead were put on trains at the
quayside and transported to Liverpool or Glasgow where they
embarked on their final passage to America.[34] While significant Jewish
communities were established in Manchester, Glasgow and Leeds, and
anti-alien sentiment was strong in those cities, it was London neighbourhoods like Whitechapel and Bethnal Green that attracted the
most attention from social and political reformers and immigration
restrictionists.[35] For these reasons, the anti-alien movement which
resulted in the passing of the 1905 Aliens Act was based, almost
entirely, on the presence of Eastern European, mostly Jewish, immigrants in the capital. The 1889 Select Committee on Alien Immigration
and the 1903 Royal Commission were both almost entirely focused on
London, and the medical evidence they requested was primarily
obtained from medical officers and other witnesses based in the city. It
is not surprising then that their recommendations in relation to arriving immigrants, while affecting other ports, were directed squarely at
the Port of London.

There was, of course, another significant immigrant group which was much more concentrated in Liverpool than London. The Irish were by far the largest immigrant group in Britain during the nineteenth century – over 800,000 by 1861 – and although they moved wherever work and opportunities arose, they predominantly settled in Liverpool, London, Glasgow and Dundee.[36] After the devastating years of the famine and the collapse of cotton and other industries, thousands flocked over the Irish Sea. But by the 1860s their numbers began to dwindle and they continued to drop in the remaining decades of the century. Thus, by the time immigration became an important issue in Britain from the late 1880s, led in no small part by developments in American immigration issues, the Irish were no longer the predominant immigrant group. Their arrival had certainly excited widespread criticism and prejudice, and the law encouraged the repatriation of thousands between 1819 and the mid-1850s. However, their presence in England, Wales and Scotland while deemed 'alien' in many respects – not least in religious terms – is perhaps better understood as an 'internal immigration.'[37] It therefore did not contribute to the rhetoric or political action that surrounded the arrival of Eastern Europeans at the end of the century, or the changes that were instituted in immigration regulations and port disease control practices at the beginning of the twentieth century; and so the migration patterns of the Irish, as well as Liverpool, for example, as an important Irish immigrant port, are not discussed in this book.

With London as the focus, then, chapter 1 begins with a review of quarantine in the nineteenth century. From early in the century the severity of quarantine restrictions was berated in Britain as 'anti-commercial, anti-social and anti-Christian'[38] and, as the century progressed, its interference with merchant shipping was 'regarded as a mere irrational derangement of commerce.'[39] It was also claimed that quarantine did not prevent disease, but rather encouraged its spread. Conversely, those who opposed quarantine also argued that traditionally 'quarantinable' diseases were not contagious and therefore could not be prevented by the physical separation of quarantine.

This chapter explores the establishment, in response to such opposition, of an alternative to quarantine – the 'English System' of port disease surveillance and control, which was more sympathetic to 'British' requirements, and sought to define a different – sanitary – construction of 'British' space. This 'System', established in 1872 with the creation of the Port Sanitary Authorities, combined the medical and sanitary regulation of shipping with 'internal' sanitary regulations – urban and rural public health. Challenging the idea that the control of imported infections created an impermeable line around the nation, whereby port health functioned as an interface between zones of sovereignty, as much as being an apparatus of prophylaxis, I argue that from its inception, the 'English System' created a more flexible border. It established a 'sanitary zone' that envisaged a wider interface of maritime space for ease of movement among British imperial ships. Much of the chapter is devoted to outlining the administration, personnel and particular duties of the two authorities. It serves to provide the structural background of infectious disease prevention at the ports, which, while elaborated in other parts of the book, sets the scene for later chapters, and adds substantially to previous scholarship relating to late-nineteenth-century port health. The subject of immigration, however, does not form part of the discussion. Unlike in the United States and elsewhere, the association between quarantine and immigration was not being made in Britain at this time. This came later. Rather, quarantine was almost exclusively and intimately connected to commerce and diplomacy, and it was administered and challenged through these channels.

Even after the establishment of the 'English System', quarantine regulations remained on the statute books until they were repealed in 1896, and they retained a significant influence over the operation of port health until the end of the century. Yet, the historiography of public health and infectious disease prevention in Britain consistently claims that quarantine was abandoned after the introduction of the Port Sanitary Authorities in 1872.[40] Chapter 1 shows how and where quarantine continued to play a role in port health, and in chapter 2 I explore why, after a preferable system had been put in place, quarantine remained for so long on the statute books.

The prevention of infectious disease at the ports – particularly the traditionally 'quarantinable' diseases of plague, yellow fever and cholera – was, with the arrival and departure of vessels from around the world, essentially an international issue. Port prophylaxis, while developed and administered domestically by British-trained medical practitioners, lawyers, politicians, clerks and so on, could not be done entirely intramurally; it required international communication and a level of internationally standardised or recognised methods of prevention. Cooperation and information sharing among maritime states, based on common concepts of disease transmission, was necessary to support the theoretical and practical foundations of the 'English System'. The second chapter focuses on the particular British approach at the International Sanitary Conferences which met frequently from 1851, and on theories of contagion in the late nineteenth century in relation to the much maligned practice of quarantine. I explore how the British and Indian colonial delegates at the conferences sought to extend the sanitary zone through strategic 'arms of the sea' such as the Suez Canal, and persuade other represented nations to abandon the costly isolation of vessels travelling between important trading centres. This chapter is therefore an examination of the interconnectedness of British ports with foreign and international relations, exploring them as part of an entangled space of negotiation with the 'outside' world, rather than places marking simply the perimeter of the 'inside' and 'domestic' realm.

The tension between conditions outside and inside the country, of foreign ports and domestic ones, and of foreign people and foreign vessels confronting British practices, is established in this chapter and is a central theme of this book. The interaction between British agendas, medical theories and practices and the policies, demands and perceptions of other countries is brought to the fore, and it becomes clear that although the 'English System' was closely associated with the internal public health and sanitary infrastructure, it was uniquely interconnected with 'foreign' health practices and policies.

The conferences have attracted growing interest among historians of global and international health; however I discuss them in chapter 2 from the unique perspective of the British and the development and application of the 'English System'. In particular, I address the presentation of British theories of cholera aetiology as they applied to the ports. These theories, while not always consistent with general trends in British disease theory, were particularly applied in relation to the economic and political exigencies of the ports as essential mechanisms within the machinery of imperial trade.[41] Although yellow fever and plague were discussed at the conferences, particularly with reference to the Mecca pilgrimages and after 1900, the primary focus of the conferences was cholera and, consequently, quarantine.[42]

Cholera's importance in Britain's response to sea-borne disease and its central role in the establishment and identity of the 'English System' is clear. It also played a critical role in immigrants becoming a growing focus of port health. Chapter 3 brings us back to 1892, the pivotal year exemplified in the incipient example of the *SS Gemma*, when cholera again threatened major European and Atlantic cities as it had so many other times since the 1830s. Generally overlooked in histories of cholera or sanitation, this was the first epidemic to test the new 'English System' and the confidence displayed by anti-quarantinists both internationally and at 'home' in the prophylactic capacities of the sanitary zone. Yet as the disease approached, even its most stalwart proponents began to lose their nerve. Their diminished faith in the surety of sanitary surveillance was linked directly to the widespread perception that Eastern European, primarily Jewish, immigrants and transmigrants (en route to America), were the prime conduits of the disease. Temporary measures, which were later incorporated into permanent Port Sanitary regulations, were aimed directly at the migrants and appeared to contradict the long-standing assertions of anti-quarantinists about movement in and through port spaces. The chapter explores how migrants came to represent a different subset within the categorisation of port diseases, and how they came to represent another notion of 'place' or 'locality' within the sanitary zone.

Key to the response to the public health 'danger' posed by migrants was the way the United States was seen to be managing the same 'threats' as they arrived at its ports. A majority of Eastern Europeans who arrived at British ports in the final decade of the nineteenth century and first decade of the next were transmigrants on their way to America. Chapter 4 explores how this directed the gaze of British public health and port authorities, as well as the increasing chorus of anti-alienists, across the Atlantic. The strict quarantine imposed against cholera vessels in New York in 1892 and the harsh medical restrictions of the 1891 Immigration Act, enforced at US entry points, received both admonition and admiration in Britain. Concern was growing that those migrants unable to gain admission to America were being returned to Britain or had decided to remain without even attempting the trans-Atlantic voyage. The increasingly medicalised categories of 'desirability' and 'undesirability' that were being created at, and were creating, the US border appeared to highlight an uncomfortable fissure in the fluidity of Britain's ports and sovereign space. This chapter examines how the elasticity of the sanitary zone, confident in its ability to protect against imported infections without the need to detain or exclude, reconciled with the growing desire among anti-alienists to adopt measures against the migrants similar to those in the United States.

The final chapter thus examines how those arguing for immigration restriction used the issue of disease control in their anti-alien narrative; how the example of American policy and practice played an important role in this part of the debate; and how immigration was positioned within, and allowed for, a differently conceptualised space at the ports. An analysis of the medical and sanitary testimony at the Royal Commission on Alien Immigration 1903 forms much of the discussion in this chapter. With the passing of the 1905 Aliens Act the space at the littoral which had previously opened up to include the domestic environment and arms of the sea that connected parts of 'Greater' Britain elasticised, contracting to define not only different and changing constructions of 'national' space but also to identify those who did and did not 'belong' within it.

The English System is therefore a history of public health and identity formation that explores the role of disease in the organisation and meaning of national boundaries. The book challenges generally held assumptions that quarantine policies in other parts of the world delineated intransigent national borders, and argues instead that the British geobody was defined as a more fluid construction. A combination of port sanitation and sanitary surveillance, known to contemporaries as the 'English System', was gradually introduced as an alternative to quarantine. With the abolition of quarantine in 1896, the importance of those disease categories based on place, which had formed its foundation and which had been adapted for the new 'English System', lessened. However, they had not collapsed but had merely been transferred. The book examines this crucial transition showing how the classification of 'foreign' and 'domestic' disease was translated, after the abolition of quarantine and during the period of mass migration, to 'foreign' and 'domestic' bodies – or the immigrant and the native population.

Notes

1 Corporation of London Records Office (CLRO), *PSCP* (July–Sept, 1892), 6 Sept. 1892.

2 Table I, *Reports and Papers on the Port and Riparian Sanitary Survey of England and Wales, 1893–4; With an Introduction by the Medical Officer of the Local Government Board* (London: HMSO, 1895) [C 7812], pp. 6–17.

3 For example, Michael Durey, *The Return of the Plague: British Society and the Cholera, 1831–2* (Dublin: Gill and Macmillan, 1979); Norman Longmate, *King Cholera: The Biography of a Disease* (London: Hamish Hamilton, 1966); R.J. Morris, *Cholera, 1832: The Social Responses to an Epidemic* (London: Croom Helm, 1976); M. Pelling, *Cholera, Fever*

and English Medicine 1825–1865 (Oxford: Oxford University Press, 1978); and William Coleman, *Yellow Fever in the North: The Methods of Early Epidemiology* (Madison: University of Wisconsin Press, 1987), pp. 139–67.

4 P. Baldwin, *Contagion and the State in Europe, 1830–1930* (Cambridge: Cambridge University Press, 1999); Graeme J. Milne, 'Institutions, Localism and Seaborne Epidemics on Late-Nineteenth-Century Tyneside,' *Northern History*, 46, 2 (2009), 261–76; Anne Hardy, 'Cholera, Quarantine and the English Preventive System, 1850–1895,' *Medical History*, 37, 3 (1993), 250–69; Jeanne L. Brand, *Doctors and the State: The British Medical Profession and Government Action in Public Health, 1870–1912* (Baltimore: Johns Hopkins University Press, 1965); G.C. Cook, *From the Greenwich Hulks to Old St Pancras: A History of Tropical Disease in London* (London: The Athlone Press, 1992); A Hardy, 'Public Health and the Expert: London Medical Officers of Health, 1856–1900', in R. MacLeod (ed.), *Government and Expertise – Specialists, Administrators and Professionals, 1860–1919* (Cambridge: Cambridge University Press, 1988), 128–42; J.C. McDonald, 'The History of Quarantine in Britain in the Nineteenth Century', *Bulletin of the History of Medicine*, xxv (1951), 22–44; D. Porter, *The History of Public Health and the Modern State* (Amsterdam: Editions Rodopi B.V., 1994).

5 Alison Bashford, *Imperial Hygiene: A Critical History of Colonialism, Nationalism and Public Health* (Hampshire and New York: Palgrave Macmillan, 2004); Alison Bashford, 'At the Border: Contagion, Immigration, Nation,' *Australian Historical Studies*, 120 (2002), 344–58; Alison Bashford (ed.), *Medicine at the Border: Disease, Globalization and Security, 1850 to the Present* (London: Palgrave Macmillan, 2006); Nayan Shah, *Contagious Divides: Epidemics and Race in San Francisco's Chinatown* (Berkeley: University of California Press, 2001); Alexandra Minna Stern, 'Buildings, Boundaries, and Blood: Medicalization and Nation-Building on the U.S.-Mexico Border, 1910–1930,' *The Hispanic American Historical Review*, 79, 1 (1999), 41–81; Howard Markel and Alexandra Minna Stern, 'Which Face? Whose Nation? Immigration, Public Health, and the Construction of Disease at America's Ports and Borders, 1891–1928,' *American Behavioral Scientist*, 42, 9 (1999), 1314–31; and David Armstrong, 'Public Health Spaces and the Fabrication of Identity,' *Sociology*, 27, 3 (1993), 393–410.

6 G. Aldermann and C. Holmes, *Outsiders and Outcasts – Essays in Honour of William J. Fishman* (London: Gerald Duckworth & Co., 1993); G. Aldermann, *London Jewry and London Politics 1889–1986* (London: Routledge, 1989); K. Collins, *Second City Jewry: The Jews of Glasgow in the Age of Expansion, 1790–1919*, 1st edn. (Glasgow: Scottish Jewish Archives, 1990); Cecil Bloom, 'The Politics of Immigration, 1881–1905', *Jewish*

Historical Studies – Transactions of the Jewish Historical Society of England, xxxiii (1992–1994), 187–214; D. Feldman, *Englishmen and Jews: Social Relations and Political Culture 1840–1914* (Yale: Yale University Press, 1994); J.A. Garrard, *The English and Immigration 1880–1910* (London, 1971); L. Gartner, *The Jewish Immigrant in England 1870–1914* (London, 1960); C. Holmes, *John Bull's Island: Immigration and British Society 1871–1971* (London: Macmillan, 1988); P. Panayi, *Immigration, Ethnicity, and Racism in Britain 1815–1945* (Manchester: Manchester University Press, 1994); K. Lunn (ed.), *Hosts, Immigrants and Minorities: Historical Responses to Newcomers in British Society, 1870–1914* (Folkestone: Dawson, 1980); Aubrey Newman (ed.), *The Jewish East End, 1840–1939* (London: Jewish Historical Society of England, 1981).

7 W. Ernst and B. Harris, *Race, Science and Medicine, 1700–1960* (London: Routledge, 1999); B. Harris, 'Anti-Alienism, Health and Social Reform in Late Victorian and Edwardian Britain', *Patterns of Prejudice,* 31 (1997), 3–34; L. Marks, 'Ethnicity, Religion and Health Care', *Social History of Medicine,* 4 (1991), 123–8; L. Marks and M. Worboys, *Migrants, Minorities and Health – Historical and Contemporary Studies* (London: Routledge, 2000).

8 Amy Fairchild, *Science at the Borders: Immigrant Medical Inspection and the Shaping of the Modern Industrial Labor Force* (Baltimore: Johns Hopkins University Press, 2003); Shah, *Contagious Divides*; Alan M. Kraut, *Silent Travelers: Germs, Genes, and the 'Immigrant Menace'* (Baltimore: The Johns Hopkins University Press, 1995); A. Kraut, 'Plagues and Prejudice: Nativism's Construction of Disease in Nineteenth- and Twentieth-Century New York City', in David Rosner (ed.), *Hives of Sickness: Public Health and Epidemics in New York City* (New Brunswick: Rutgers University Press, 1995), 65–90; A.E. Birn, 'Six Seconds Per Eyelid: The Medical Inspection of Immigrants at Ellis Island, 1892–1914', *Dynamics,* 17 (1997), 281–316; D. Hoerder and H. Rössler, *Distant Magnets: Expectations and Realities in the Immigration Experience 1840–1930* (New York: Holmes & Meire Publishers, Inc., 1993); H. Markel, 'Cholera, Quarantines, and Immigration Restriction: The View from Johns Hopkins, 1892', *Bulletin of the History of Medicine,* 67 (1993), 691–5; H. Markel, '"Knocking Out the Cholera": Cholera, Class, and Quarantines in New York City, 1892', *Bulletin of the History of Medicine,* 69 (1995), 420–57; H. Markel, *Quarantine! East European Jewish Immigrants and the New York City Epidemics of 1892* (Baltimore and London: Johns Hopkins University Press, 1997); H. Markel, and A.M. Stern, 'All Quiet on the Third Coast: Medical Inspections of Immigrants in Michigan', *Public Health Reports,* 114 (1999), 178–82; J. Parascandola, 'Doctors at the Gate: PHS at Ellis Island', *Public Health Reports,* 113 (1998), 83–6; C.E. Rosenberg, *The Cholera Years – The United States in 1832, 1849, and 1866,* With a New Foreword (Chicago: University of Chicago Press, 1987); R.T. Solis-Cohen, 'The Exclusion of Aliens from the United States for Physical Defects', *Bulletin of the History of Medicine,* 21 (1947), 33–50.

9 Markel, *Quarantine!*, p. 5.

10 *The Lancet*, Feb. 18, 1893, p. 375; see also, for example, 'Destitute Jews', *The Lancet*, Sept. 17, 1887, p. 599; *BMJ*, Sept. 10–Oct. 15, 1892; 'The Immigration of Undesirable Aliens', *BMJ*, Aug. 22, 1903, pp. 423–4; *The Times*, Nov. 6, 1901, p. 12f; 'Trachoma among Aliens', *The Lancet*, June 3, 1905, p. 1525.

11 Hardy, 'Cholera'; see also chapter 1.

12 Krista Maglen, '"The First Line of Defense:" British Quarantine and the Port Sanitary Authorities in the Nineteenth Century,' *Social History of Medicine*, 15 (2002), 413–28; also, Milne, 'Institutions.'

13 Hardy, 'Cholera', p. 268.

14 *Ibid.*, p. 263.

15 Bashford, *Imperial Hygiene*, p. 123.

16 See for example, Hastings Donnan and Thomas M. Wilson, *Borders: Frontiers of Identity, Nation and State* (Oxford and New York: Berg, 1999), p. 132.

17 Fairchild, *Science at the Borders*, p. 16.

18 Bryan S. Turner, 'Social Fluids: Metaphors and Meanings of Society,' *Body and Society*, 9, 1 (2003), 1–10, p. 3.

19 Referenced in Ann Laura Stoler, 'Sexual Affronts and Racial Frontiers: European Ideas and the Cultural Politics of Exclusion in Colonial Southeast Asia', 'in Cooper, Frederick and Stoler, Ann Laura (eds), *Tensions of Empire: Colonial Cultures in a Bourgeois World* (Berkeley: University of California Press, 1997), 198–237, p. 199.

20 Sarah Palmer, 'Ports,' in Daunton, Martin J. (ed.), *The Cambridge Urban History of Britain, Vol. III, 1840–1950* (Cambridge: Cambridge University Press, 2000), 133–50, p. 134.

21 *Ibid.*

22 Linda Colley, 'Britishness and Otherness: An Argument', *Journal of British Studies*, 31, 4 (1992), 309–29; and Hugh Kearney, 'Four Nations History in Perspective,' in Brocklehurst, Helen and Phillips, Robert (eds), *History, Nationhood and the Question of Britain* (London: Palgrave Macmillan, 2004), 10–19.

23 Roxanne Lynn Doty, 'Immigration and National Identity: Constructing the Nation,' *Review of International Studies*, 22, 3 (1996), 235–55, p. 242.

24 Keith Robbins, 'The "British Space": World-Empire-Continent-Nation-Region-Locality: A Historiographical Problem,' *History Compass*, 7, 1 (2009), 66–94, p. 69.

25 Ian Convery, John Welshmand and Alison Bashford, 'Where Is the Border?: Screening for Tuberculosis in the United Kingdom and Australia, 1950–2000,' in Bashford (ed.), *Medicine at the Border*, pp. 97–115.

26 John Welshman, 'Compulsion, Localism, and Pragmatism: The Micro-Politics of Tuberculosis Screening in the United Kingdom, 1950–1965,' *Social History of Medicine*, 19, 2 (2006), 295–312, p, 308.

27 *Ibid.*, p. 311.
28 Robbins, 'British Space,' p. 73; and, Jan Rüger, 'Nation, Empire and Navy: Identity Politics in the United Kingdom, 1887–1914,' *Past and Present*, 185 (2004), 159–87, p. 168.

    For contemporary use of the term 'English System' see, for example, W. Collingridge, 'The Milroy Lectures: On Quarantine', Part 2, *BMJ*, March 20, 1897, p. 713.
29 Patrick Zylberman, 'Civilizing the State: Borders, Weak States and International Health in Modern Europe,' in Bashford, *Medicine at the Border*, pp. 21–40, 32–5.
30 Owen Lattimore, *Studies in Frontier History: Collected Papers, 1928–1958* (Oxford: Oxford University Press, 1962), p. 113.
31 Previously held at the CLRO.
32 Palmer, 'Ports,' p. 140.
33 Paul Knepper, 'British Jews and the Radicalisation of Crime in the Age of Empire,' *British Journal of Criminology*, 47, 1 (2007), 61–79, p. 63.
34 Nicholas J. Evans, 'Indirect Passage from Europe: Transmigration via the UK, 1836–1914,' *Journal for Maritime Research*, 3, 1 (2001), 70–84, p. 71.
35 Lloyd P. Gartner, *American and British Jews in the Age of the Great Migration* (London and Portland, OR: Vallentine Mitchell, 2009), p. 59.
36 Leo Lucassen, *The Immigrant Threat: The Integration of Old and New Migrants in Western Europe Since 1850* (Chicago: University of Illinois Press, 2005), p. 30.
37 David Feldman, 'Was the Nineteenth Century a Golden Age for Immigrants? The Changing Articulation of National, Local and Voluntary Controls,' in Andreas Fahrmeir, Oliver Faron and Patrick Weil (eds), *Migration Control in the North Atlantic World: The Evolution of State Practices in Europe and the United States from the French Revolution to the Inter-War Period* (New York and London: Berghahn Books, 2003), 167–77, p. 170.
38 *Hansard*, 1825, vol. XII, p. 993, quoted in McDonald, 'The History of Quarantine', p. 26.
39 *BMJ*, Oct 8, 1887, p. 778.
40 See note 5.
41 On general trends in British disease theory see Michael Worboys, *Spreading Germs: Disease Theories and Medical practice in Britain, 1865–1900* (Cambridge: Cambridge University Press, 2000).
42 W.F. Bynum, 'Policing Hearts of Darkness: Aspects of the International Sanitary Conferences', *History and Philosophy of the Life Sciences*, 15 (1993), 421–34, p. 428.

1

'The first line of defence...'

The interconnectedness of distant and disparate parts of the world, which had grown with European new imperialism and the speed of steam travel in the late nineteenth century, brought new concerns about the corresponding transit of disease. Places, spaces and people, once separated by vast oceans or endless steppes were now brought into much closer proximity, while new environments created through changing patterns of urbanisation and industry, through conflict or colonisation, created fertile settings for the emergence and spread of old and new infections. Arresting the advance of these threats traditionally meant intercepting and detaining, through the use of quarantines, the ships and trains, passengers and seamen which facilitated this connectivity.

As well as being used for defending the population against the invasion of foreign diseases, quarantine facilitated other state functions. Importantly, it reinforced bounded notions of the nation during a period of national consolidation and used medical categories to classify people and spaces as constituent or not of those nations. As Alison Bashford has argued, 'Quarantine, more than any other government technology *is* the drawing and policing of boundaries. Quarantine and nationalism imply each other because both are about the creation of spaces.'[1]

By contrast, in Britain the relationship between quarantine and nation looked considerably different. From the early decades of the nineteenth century the use of maritime quarantine for the interception of 'exotic' disease began to lose favour among a growing number of both medical practitioners and politicians. Rather than strengthening quarantine lines in the dual effort of controlling disease and policing the border, arguments were made for its termination in favour of more moderate alternatives that permitted the functioning of a more flexible border. The policy of isolation and exclusion which quarantine demanded – prohibiting people and goods on board infected vessels from any intercourse with the shore for up to thirty days[2] – was considered to be in conflict with British liberal economic principles. As George Buchanan, Britain's Chief Medical Officer from 1879 to 1892, declared,

> England imposes no restrictions upon intercourse between one and another community – town and town, nation and nation ... She would dispense, in land and sea traffic alike, with those detentions known as quarantines, having found them in practice to result rather in hazardous concealments and evasions than in any effectual exclusion of [disease].[3]

The apparent inability of quarantine to prevent the importation of disease and its obvious interference with maritime trade led to a general and growing resistance towards it, which was manifest from the early decades of the century through to its last.

Furthermore, quarantine could not function in the same way as a nation-marking structure in Britain where the national border was not as simple as the geographical line around the island(s). It differed significantly from the model suggested by Bashford for Australia whereby 'A national maritime quarantine "line" was created, which *was* the border of the new nation ... Part of the effect of quarantine was the imagining of Australia as an island-nation, in which "island" stood for "immunity"'. Questions about the spatial 'imagining' of Britain, let alone issues of 'Britishness' and British national identity, were more complicated than the geographical boundaries of the 'British Isles': Were Ireland and the Irish part of the same geo-body as England, for example? And how were the numerous parts of Britain's empire to fit within defined boundaries of 'British' space? Could white settler colonies, such as Australia and Canada, be included in the 'British' geo-body, while India, with the greatest maritime connections to Britain, was placed outside the drawing of national quarantine lines?[4] In exploring this idea of a more expansive, but clearly ill-defined, idea of 'Britain', the eminent Cambridge historian John Seeley wrote in his enormously popular book *The Expansion of Britain* (1883), 'our Empire is not an Empire at all in the ordinary sense of the word. It does not consist of a congeries of nations held together by force, but in the main one nation, as much as if it were no Empire but an ordinary state.'[5] Seeley further expounded on the idea of a 'Greater Britain' which had been used variously to describe the unity of the empire as a whole, or its white settler colonies, or any predominantly English-speaking country.[6] In Seeley's influential book it was employed to refer collectively to 'Englishmen beyond the seas', but did not extend to the 'native races' that made up the vast population of his notion of 'Greater Britain' as an (extra) 'ordinary state'. Clearly then, to attempt delineate 'British' space, in Seeley's model or any other contemporary permutation, was not possible using the blunt edge of quarantine.

The openness of Britain, in any of its permutations (island, United Kingdom, empire) related to the movement of both goods and people, and so the same instincts that rejected quarantine also rejected restrictions to immigration. As the century drew to a close, Britain began increasingly to distinguish itself in its commitment to the openness of its borders in relation to both. However, immigration to Britain from anywhere other than Ireland was minimal for most of the nineteenth century and was equally unimportant politically or as a policy issue. It therefore did not enter into conversations about the porousness of any of the manifestations of 'Britain'. Quarantine, on the other hand, became deeply problematic for any such consideration.

More accommodating of the complicated form of Britain and useful for helping to define a broader biological border 'zone' was what became known as the English System of disease prevention, administered by the Port Sanitary Authorities. This system, established in 1872, allowed for much greater freedom of movement into and through British ports than quarantine did, requiring that only ships that arrived with visible signs of disease on board should be disinfected, and the sick removed to an isolation hospital. Anyone else who appeared to be healthy should be allowed to disembark and enter into the community, where they would be monitored by local medical officers. Unlike under the quarantine system, Bills of Health[7] (upon which pratique, or free entry to the port, was granted) were issued on the basis of the presence of disease on board a vessel, not based on the presence of disease in its departure port. The English System also, importantly, combined the medical and sanitary regulation of shipping with 'internal' sanitary regulations – urban and rural public health. So, rather than the control of imported infections creating an impermeable line around the nation, whereby port health functioned as an interface between zones of sovereignty as much as being an apparatus of prophylaxis, the English System created a more equivocal border. It operated in a different spatial milieu defined by sanitary reform, which, as Michelle Allen has shown, 'was necessarily a spatial phenomenon' concerned with the physical environments and geographies of cities, and the people and places connected to them.[8] The geo-body was not to be defined therefore at the littoral, but by networks of sanitary norms and spaces.

Quarantine in the nineteenth century

In an important annual lecture at the Royal College of Physicians in London, established by the quarantine reformer Gavin Milroy, the second and long-serving Port Medical Officer of Health for London, William Collingridge, defined quarantine in the following terms:

> [Quarantine comprises] ... preventative measures designed to prevent the importation of disease into a country by means of maritime commerce, it may be defined as 'the enforced detention and segregation of vessels arriving in a port, together with all persons and things on board, believed to be infected with the poison of certain epidemic diseases for specific periods'. ... The essential point of quarantine at its earliest inception up to its fully developed existence at the present day is that it estimates the danger, and thereupon the precautions to be taken, according to the state of health of the port from whence the vessel has arrived, and has no reference to the condition as regards health or sickness of the vessel and its inhabitants.[9]

While quarantine did, in fact, respond to the presence of 'sickness' on board a vessel, often resulting in protracted detention, its response to so-called 'suspected' vessels was a defining feature. Suspected ships were those which had proceeded from an 'infected' port or which had had some contact with infection. No cases or suspected cases of the disease on board needed to be manifest in order for quarantine to be imposed.

What has historically distinguished 'quarantine' from 'isolation' is that the latter is concerned with the removal and detention of individuals who have displayed the signs and symptoms of disease. Quarantine, on the other hand, calls for the incarceration of sick and healthy alike, as well as goods and vessels. It not merely seeks to separate cases of illness from the broader community but requires the exclusion from society of those people and things that have potentially been contaminated through any connection with sources of disease. Thus, chains of connectivity with people, places or spaces thought to present a risk are assessed, rather than individual well-being. For these reasons, quarantine has been both feared and resented. It has been feared because it could mean that healthy passengers may be detained along with infected patients, and were historically confined together on board a vessel or incarcerated in a land-based quarantine station. And, it has been resented for the time and relinquished freedoms demanded of healthy individuals, as well as the costly delays enforced on travel, transportation and commerce.

By the early nineteenth century, the latter of these vexations had taken over as the primary concern associated with quarantine in Britain. Shipping was an essential instrument in Britain's growing empire, generating enormous wealth and securing British naval and imperial dominance. Quarantine could create enormous problems for maritime trade, potentially adding, by the turn of the nineteenth century, over thirty days onto the duration of a journey. During a month of detention another trip might have been completed (depending on where the ship had travelled from), perishable goods may have decayed, if not been destroyed, and a hefty quarantine duty would need to have been paid. The imposition of quarantine was derided as 'a barbarous encumbrance, interrupting commerce, obstructing international intercourse, periling life, and wasting, and worse than wasting, large sums of public money'.[10]

However, as I discuss in chapter 2, the fundamental principle upon which quarantine rested was the idea of contagion and, until at least the mid-nineteenth century, this essentially outweighed the grievances uttered against the cost. If a disease was believed to be communicated from one person to another, the only way to stop it was to 'break chains of transmission, interrupting the circulation of carriers by means of cordons, quarantines and sequestration'.[11] By isolating or excluding the infection, it could be excluded from a community. The traditional period of forty days initially would have covered the time needed to ensure that the disease was neither incubating nor still extant in any virulent form. With changing understanding of different diseases, this period of confinement was reduced by the end of the eighteenth century to twenty to thirty days. Thus, while a disease was considered to be contagious, quarantine was the only method that could be applied against it. Yet, if a disease was not considered to be contagious, but rather was seen to be generated and contracted by people through some means other than person-to-person (or object-to-person), quarantine had little use. Aetiological theories which maintained a causal relationship between disease and locality, environment and 'filth', and that grew out of eighteenth-century ideas linking climate with disease, therefore held great appeal and flourished in the anti-quarantine milieu of nineteenth-century Britain.[12] Not only did these so-called anti-contagionist theories support Chadwickian sanitary reform and the viability of the heavy-handed Poor Law,[13] they also served as a useful tool in arguments opposing the institution and practice of quarantine.[14] However, it was not until the middle of the century that anti-contagionist theories began significantly to threaten the conceptual basis upon which quarantine had been built. Until then quarantine maintained a secure place in legislation and was a prophylactic strategy relied upon around coastal Britain for protection against invading infections.

The first quarantine act of the nineteenth century (40 Geo. III. c.80) passed in 1800 called for the building of a lazaretto (maritime quarantine station) on Chetney Hill near Dartford and required 'that the cost of Quarantine be borne by incoming ships.'[15] The building of the lazaretto was unduly prolonged due to a variety of practical problems, and within a few years of its completion it was found to be ineffectual.[16] Yet, smaller quarantine stations were maintained in the major ports, and a special lazaretto was constructed at Milford as 'a Foul Bill [of Health] station – for ships to the western part of the Kingdom'. Another 'Foul Bill station' in Liverpool served the 'eastern part'. Goods which arrived on an infected ship were aired on deck from three to six days before being removed to the lazaretto.[17] There, bales and packages were opened and the process of airing was continued for up to a further 40 days. Passengers and crew were required to remain on board the vessel for up to 30 days after all the goods were removed. The whole process, for a ship arriving with a Foul Bill of Health, could take up to sixty to sixty-five days.[18]

The main opponent of quarantine in the early years of the nineteenth century was Charles Maclean (1788–1824). Maclean was a physician who had been employed for most of his career as a surgeon with the East India Company and the Levant Company, and lectured to the East India Company on the diseases of hot climates.[19] He was convinced that plague, the primary target at which quarantine measures were aimed, was not contagious but rather 'dependant on atmospheric influences'. During the period 1817–24 he published a number of medical books and pamphlets in opposition to quarantine, such as *Evils of Quarantine Laws and Non-Existence of Pestilential Contagion Deduced from the Phenomena of the Plague of the Lavant, the Yellow Fever of Spain and the Cholera Morbus of Asia* (London, 1824).[20]

In them he argued, providing a neat summary of anti-quarantine grievances, that quarantine was 'really the cause of 19/20 of all epidemics by
enforcing confinement in pestilential air; producing concealment of
the disease, desertion of the sick, and deadly terror. Quarantines were
amoral, ineffective and the source of enormous gratuitous expenses
and vexation.'[21]

Responding to an increase in this kind of criticism, the government
appointed a Select Committee in 1819, with not a little of Maclean's
influence, to 'investigate the validity of the doctrine of contagion in
plague.'[22] The Committee concluded that plague was indeed contagious, passing directly from person to person, and that therefore there
was no reason to question the principles upon which quarantine was
based. The subject was revisited again five years later when another
Select Committee met to consider how foreign trade might be improved.
Its members pronounced that as quarantine and contagion were insep-
arable, all information on the subject, as prudence dictated, should be
taken from medical witnesses with known contagionist leanings. Not
surprisingly, they all concluded that the present quarantine regulations were sufficient and that quarantine was necessary for preventing
the import of epidemic disease. Part of their report is worth quoting at
some length:

> [The] Committee have called before them several medical men of
> eminence, whose opinions appeared the best calculated to assist
> them in pursuing the object of their inquiry, and coming to a satis-
> factory conclusion. In making their selection ... they have confined
> themselves to those whose attention had not only been directed to
> this subject, but whose opinions were understood to be in favour of
> the received doctrine of Contagion: their reason for this was, that it
> being their object to ascertain the degree of relaxation in the present
> regulations that might be safely adopted, consistently with the expe-
> rience of danger, no advantage could arise from having recourse to
> the opinions of those who entirely disbelieve the possibility of Con-
> tagion, and considered every precaution to guard against it mis-
> placed and unnecessary.[23]

While the Committee was somewhat critical of a few of the European
methods and regulations for quarantine, it recommended a consolidation of all previous quarantine legislation into a single act and the
enforcement of twenty-one days detention for all quarantinable vessels.[24] A Bill was drawn up which embodied the recommendations.
Maclean petitioned the government for the complete rejection of

this and all quarantine regulations, arguing that they were 'without an object, as an absolutely demonstrated evil, as a code eminently anti-commercial, anti-social, and anti-Christian'.[25] He and other anti-quarantinists vehemently objected to the Bill on the grounds that neither the 1819 nor the 1824 Select Committee had taken evidence from any anti-contagionists, despite the fact that this way of thinking was continuing to attract the support of a growing number of medical men. Nevertheless, the government was determined to err on the side of caution and, despite the objections, concluded that it was more prudent to continue with the Bill. It was argued that in terms of trade, when the rest of Europe, if not the world, were firmly in favour of quarantine, Britain could ill afford the loss of trade incurred if her ports were deemed dangerous because of an absence of quarantine laws. Indeed, during the deliberations some Mediterranean countries had begun to impose precautionary quarantines on British vessels regardless of 'infected' or 'suspect' status. The President of the Board of trade cautioned that 'we had brought on our commerce a severe infliction, in consequence of the discussion of this question'.[26]

The Bill carried through both Houses, and in 1825 the Quarantine Act (6 Geo. III c.78) was passed.[27] The Act applied to all vessels that arrived from any port infected with '*Plague or other infectious disease or distemper highly dangerous to the health of His Majesty's subjects*' as well as '*the Yellow Fever or other highly infectious distemper [which] prevails on the Continent of America, or in the West Indies*'.[28] It also placed quarantine within the authority of the Privy Council, directing the Customs Service to perform the functions of the Act, and it was not long before the new law was put to the test.

For two years between 1830 and 1832 western Europe was confronted with its first epidemic of 'Asiatic Cholera' – the 'exotic' disease originating from India – which had been brought west with growing European mercantile interaction with the Indian Ocean. It flourished in the expanding urban environment of industrialisation and in the exceptionally warm summer of 1831.[29] In April of that year, after learning that cholera had arrived in St Petersburg and was slowly pushing westward, and in anticipation of the approaching disease, the Admiralty ordered that a strict quarantine be imposed on all ships arriving from foreign ports.[30] By June the Privy Council provided for a temporary inclusion of cholera within the existing quarantine laws and a consultative Central Board of Health was established to oversee its implementation. The Privy Council then issued regulations in October 1831 in which strict quarantine was to be imposed on both sea and land.

However, on 9 October the first case of cholera was reported in Sunderland.[31] Not only did the disease claim thousands of lives in its first great scourge of Britain, but its ferocity appeared almost unprecedented. Unlike other epidemic diseases such as tuberculosis, which according to Richard Evans spread 'at a leisurely pace', cholera whirled through towns and cities, and through the bodies of its victims, with devastating effect.[32] Its onset was rapid and violent, horrifying Victorian sensibilities, with the possibility of sudden and uncontrollable vomiting and diarrhoea. Within hours victims could descend into grave illness, becoming cadaverous, shrivelled and displaying the characteristic blue complexion brought on by extreme dehydration. Their bodies were racked by agonising spasms, after which most victims would fall into a state of collapse and semi-consciousness, speaking, if at all, in a rasping whisper, and finally, in about fifty per cent of cases, dying. The whole process could occur in as little as five hours, but more commonly endured for three to four days.

In an effort to protect the population from the horrors of this new disease, local boards of health were instructed to carry out the provisions of the Quarantine Act inland from the ports and record all instances of infection. Infected towns were quarantined, and individual houses were marked with signs of 'CAUTION' or 'SICK'. The quarantine period was not less than twenty days, and applied to the sick, those who had been in contact with them and those who had any ill-timed bouts of quite harmless diarrhoea. All incoming ships from foreign ports were also placed in quarantine for not less than twenty days. Infected or suspected ships were moored to floating lazarettos, where all goods on board were aired and treated with chlorine fumes; passengers and crew were forced to remain on board. The sick and the healthy were confined together, often without any medical assistance.[33] Quarantines were even imposed on intra-national shipping, so that vessels arriving in London from some Northern ports, such as Sunderland and Newcastle, were detained for fifteen days in an attempt to arrest the spread of disease.[34] Although a variety of problems were associated with the quarantine regime, most people placed a great reliance on it for assuring the safety of the British population. The popular *London*

Medical Gazette, which represented the conservative voice of the medical profession,[35] avowed:

> True, [quarantines] are injurious to trade, but what of that? The profits of the merchant must give place to the safety of the public: true they are detrimental to the revenue; but surely it would be better, if need be, to levy a tax upon the purses of liege subjects than upon their lives. Besides, the period of doubt cannot last long: if the disease come, why then farewell to further quarantine, at least by sea: if it be kept out, then the measureless benefit of its exclusion will reconcile the most prejudiced and discontented to the temporary inconvenience.[36]

Yet, despite the extent and rigours of quarantine measures which were put in place, cholera did arrive on British shores and continued to spread inland throughout 1832. This was partly due to the fact that smuggling had increased with a gusto to match the rigidity of the quarantine regulations, and also because, particularly during this first epidemic, the disease was so little understood. The *coup de main* of the new disease, along with its mysterious aetiology, terrified the public and sent the medical profession into a frenzy of observing and theorising. As the disease appeared to follow neither the 'normal' paths of human intercourse nor any patterns of climate, methods of prevention for plague were applied.[37]

However, the containment of cholera was largely unsuccessful, and during 1831–32 it was estimated that 30,900 people died from the disease in England.[38] It was this failure of quarantine procedures to protect the British public from the importation of cholera during the first epidemic and those of the following two decades which encouraged a more widespread opposition to the system. The sacrifices required by quarantine had not been compensated with safety, liberating ideas which explored possible alternatives to disease prevention at the ports. This, combined with the strength of developing sanitary reforms from the 1840s, prompted some precocious suggestions in a report written after the 1848–49 cholera epidemic to extend sanitary methods to the ports:

> It does not appear that the Quarantine has been of any avail in cholera ... A sanatory [sic] maritime police is therefore indispensable; into which it would be advantageous to convert all the quarantine officers of Europe. The futile, superstitious practices of the lazarettos are as contemptible in the eyes of science as they are injurious to commerce.[39]

Displaying an unequivocal opposition to quarantine, the General Board of Health's 1849 *Report on Quarantine* contributed to growing support for anti-contagionist theories in respect to quarantine. Margaret Pelling has emphasised the importance of this report in noting its effect in 'arousing the latent opposition of the medical profession' to quarantine.[40] Co-written by founding sanitarians the Earl of Carlisle, Lord Ashley, Edwin Chadwick and Thomas Southwood-Smith, the report set about proving through accumulated 'evidence' and 'experience' that not only were 'epidemic' diseases not contagious but also that quarantine had failed to prevent imported infection. It sought to reveal 'whether quarantine can prevent the extension of epidemic diseases, whatever may be their nature, whether contagious or not'.[41] Essentially, it was a manifesto on the non-contagious nature of epidemic disease, and the subsequent importance and superiority of sanitary methods over the purportedly misinformed and ineffectual practice of quarantine.

Yet, despite these sentiments, quarantine remained in wide use for the reception of cholera patients, and it continued to display its devastating deficiencies. In 1852, the prominent epidemiologist and compiler of statistics for the Registrar General, William Farr, put together a *Report on the Mortality of Cholera in England, 1848–1849*. In it he noted a disparity in the morbidity and mortality of the 1831–32 and 1848–49 epidemics. The significant increase in the late 1840s epidemic was, however, not attributed to any relaxation of quarantine but, as support for more miasmatic theories of disease aetiology grew, to the worsening of conditions in industrial towns and cities.[42] This focus on 'miasma' – an ambiguous term generally meaning disease poisons found in the noxious air associated with overcrowding, dampness, lack of ventilation and drainage, and emanating from all kinds of filth – and the role it was attributed in the cause of cholera served anti-quarantinists well.[43]

But little was still known about the cause of cholera. By the late 1850s the waterborne theory was given some support, others favoured miasmatic theories, while numerous variations on these were also used to account for its transmission.[44] Meanwhile, quarantine was losing widespread support, both because of its failure to prevent the 1832, 1848 and 1854 epidemics – 'it does not appear that the Quarantine has been of any avail in cholera', Farr's report announced[45] – and its incompatibility with Britain's commitment to the ideology of *laissez faire* and desire to protect the unfettered passage of its merchant and naval vessels. The latter, particularly, distinguished Britain from other European countries in its increasing rejection of quarantine and its formulating of alternative preventative measures against the disease.

Even so, as the 1824 Select Committee on Quarantine had noted, Britain was obliged to conform somewhat with international maritime quarantine requirements, even while it began to assemble different ways of thinking about port protections. Throughout the 1850s and 1860s the threat of cholera was increasingly responded to with sanitary improvements and growing professionalisation and legislation in the area of public health.[46] By the mid-1860s, considerable advancements had been made in the general sanitation and sanitary organisation of London and other major cities. However, in 1866 epidemic cholera struck Europe once again, this time originating in Egypt. This epidemic was the last to have any significant effect in Britain – killing seven in every 10,000 of the population[47] – and demonstrated that British defences were lacking in two key areas: the cleanliness of its cities and the health regulation of shipping.[48]

Further enquiries into the efficacy of employing quarantine for cholera in the 1860s began to recommend that alternative strategies for arresting the progress of the disease be sought. For example, in 1861 the 'Social Science Quarantine Committee' submitted a report, published by the Board of Trade, recommending, importantly, that when a vessel arrived in a port and had been inspected by the Quarantine Medical Officer, any cases of illness should be removed to hospital but 'the healthy should not be detained'.[49] Similarly, in 1868 a deputation of leading medical men appealed to the Privy Council to find an alternative to quarantine, claiming that not only had it caused great 'inconvenience' but that it had failed to protect against any epidemic of cholera since 1832.[50]

In the meantime, the development of the country's national sanitary system of public health provision and monitoring had, from the 1850s, gotten well underway, and Medical Officers of Health had overseen the public health of a number of local areas since the passing of the 1848 Public Health Act. However, the role of the Medical Officers of Health whose districts touched upon rivers, ports and harbours was, from the late 1860s, beginning to be questioned. These were brought to light at the 1869 Royal Sanitary Commission where it was revealed that ships lying within a harbour were 'considered under no sanitary authority'.[51] J.R. Slebbing, the Medical Officer of Health for Southampton, a major trade and migration port for North and South

America and Southern Africa, informed the Commission of particular difficulties associated with cholera prevention. He explained that because the disease did not fall strictly within the wording and possible remit of the Quarantine Act – being neither plague nor yellow fever – the landing of cases of cholera had proved to be highly problematic. The issue lay in the fact that while a cholera case was on board a vessel within the harbour it was not immediately within the boundaries of the Custom Service, not being strictly 'quarantinable', or either a sanitary authority or a parish or borough. It was therefore very unclear who bore responsibility for its prevention and the costs incurred. At the same time, if the case was landed within the quarantine period, international agreements required that any ship subsequently sailing from Southampton would not be granted a clean Bill of Health.[52] As Slebbing explained, the option to quarantine was unavoidable but undesirable:

> the moment we land a person with cholera we place every ship from Southampton in quarantine all over the world, and very seriously affect the packet service of the country... [However], you cannot put them in quarantine; it is a very unsafe thing to land the passengers, and it is a serious thing to keep them out in the water with the germs of the disease on board.[53]

Slebbing's account of Southampton could be repeated at numerous other international ports throughout Britain, which shared the problems inherent to there being no official means for ensuring a thorough medical examination of each ship, and also no means for dealing with any illness found on board which was not specified under the Quarantine Act. Vessels could be detained by Customs only if a case of plague or yellow fever was suspected, or if a cholera epidemic threatened, and a General Order had been issued with the specific intent of quarantining vessels which arrived from infected ports. Otherwise, the Customs Quarantine Service was not responsible. Yet, while they remained in the 'in-between' space of the port, ships infected with non-quarantinable diseases – categorised as 'indigenous' diseases – also lay beyond the jurisdiction of the local urban sanitary authorities and the local poor law parishes or boroughs. The Harbour Commission, which governed various aspects of the Port of Southampton, like similar bodies in other ports, did not employ a medical member or officer and its 'jurisdiction in sanitary matters would be a very questionable thing'.[54] Thus, in effect no authority had jurisdiction over or responsibility for cases of non-quarantinable disease, including cholera, which was brought on board a ship into a British port.

Cholera fell into an 'in-between' category – neither 'indigenous' nor 'exotic' – and starkly illuminated the ambiguities of maritime disease control at British ports. A fissure had formed between the exclusionary distance of quarantine, which was largely unwanted, and Britain's domestic public health mechanisms, leaving the ports suspended in between. Beyond plague or yellow fever, which remained firmly under the control of quarantine, 'indigenous' disease and the anomalous status of cholera were marooned in an equivocal category of health management while at the ports. The sanitary reforms brought in by the passage of the 1848 Public Health Act had been as much about urban management and the control of pauperism as they were about the elimination of disease,[55] dealing with disease and its causes as social problems, stemming from within the population and local environments. There was little room, therefore, for the consideration of 'indigenous' diseases, such as nebulous 'fevers', which arrived on board ships from abroad; these did not fit within the conceptualisation of disease that drove public health and sanitary planning. Quarantine, regardless of its unpopularity, took care of the problem of 'exotic' disease, arriving from distant shores, and sanitary infrastructure and policing took care of 'indigenous' maladies which arose from the noxious gasses of decomposing matter in Britain's towns and cities. However, during the middle decades of the century, any disease other than plague or yellow fever that arrived at the ports slipped into a space that was essentially undefined, and certainly unprotected.

Responding to this problem, the 1869 Sanitary Royal Commission recommended that any urban or rural sanitary authorities adjacent to a harbour should extend their powers and those of their representatives to act 'for sanitary purposes in the harbour' – thus extending sanitary control outwards from the local and domestic sphere.[56] It also recommended that the sanitary authorities which incorporated the harbours should work cooperatively with the Quarantine Service and attend to ships which carried on board cases of infectious disease not touched by the Quarantine Act, in other words, 'indigenous' disease.[57] These recommendations were incorporated into the Public Health Act of 1872, which established a comprehensive system of urban and rural sanitary districts, each with a Medical Officer of Health, which covered the entire country. Among these districts were port and riparian sanitary districts to which the local authorities appointed sanitary and medical officers – the Port Medical Officers of Health.

The Port Sanitary Authorities and the application of sanitary methods of prevention at the ports thus became the basis of the English System. This system and the professional groups established for it were unique and distinctive and were developed both as a means of providing a more comprehensive system for the reception of infected vessels and as an alternative to quarantine. Its particular identification and naming as an English System was not insignificant or accidental. This, it was important for all to know, was a preventative mechanism that would define not only 'English' – more accurately 'British' – port health, but also 'English' (or 'British') space. It would mark a sanitary, spatial and political category that was both distinctive and authoritative and, it was hoped, remarkably 'English'.

Making an English System

The Sanitary Royal Commission and the 1872 Public Health Act provided the legal requirement and foundations for the expansion of the sanitary system outwards to the ports and sought to rectify the deficits in 'indigenous' disease control. Looking back in 1887, Richard Thorne Thorne, Britain's medical delegate to numerous International Sanitary Conferences, explained:

> But what is our alternative system? Having deliberately abandoned the system of quarantine,[58] we began, many years ago, to organise the system of medical inspection with isolation. The medical inspection comes first into operation on our coasts ... The medical inspection is thus followed by isolation of the sick. Unlike a quarantine system, this process does not interfere with the healthy, or expose them to risk by herding them together with the sick, but the names of the healthy and the places of their destination are taken down, and the medical officer of health of the districts in question are informed of the impending arrivals. This part of our system has been named our first line of defence ...[59]

This first line of defence brought together the independently operating, localised authorities which had offered assorted responses to cases of imported 'indigenous' disease prior to 1872. Although remaining within local administration, disease and sanitary control of the ports was brought under the central, standard agency of the Local Government

Board. For example, before 1872 a selection of independently operating *ad hoc* authorities protected the Port of London from the introduction of non-quarantinable sea-borne infectious diseases. These included: the Thames Shipping Inspection Committee, representing riverside parishes in the prevention of cholera; forty-six individual riverside authorities; the Thames Conservancy; and Her Majesty's Customs Service. Similar joint authorities operated in other ports around the country although no organised system consolidated the methods of prevention practised around Britain's coastline.[60]

The 1872 Public Health Act created Port Sanitary Districts and expanded the administration of pre-existing local sanitary authorities (urban or rural) or created new Port Sanitary Authorities for the public health of the ports.[61] The effect was to standardise the approach to port prophylaxis and, as Anne Hardy has pointed out, bring a 'systematic supervision of entry to the country'.[62] Generally, the port authorities were modelled on the existing structures of urban and rural sanitary districts. Very often, in smaller ports the Port Medical Officer became an extension of the role and duties of the position of Medical Officer of Health for the local sanitary district. As the busiest ports, London and Liverpool were exceptional in that the Port Medical Officer was employed on a full-time basis. In London, due to the size and heterogeneous nature of the business of the port, various medical and sanitary officers were employed to oversee the health of the port.

What the creation of the Port Sanitary Authorities attempted to do was to push outward the control exerted over the homes and bodies of the poor in Britain's towns and cities to the in-between spaces of the ports and the ships that entered them. The new dispensation would integrate the ports into the landscape of the internal and local sanitary environments, by attempting to standardise the way corporeal and spatial health were regulated at the littoral. This new English System would locate British sovereignty in more fluid spatial terms than the unambiguous line of quarantine, but would demonstrate unmistakably the boundaries of 'Englishness' through sanitary regulation, beginning to define categories of 'inclusion' and 'exclusion' through cleanliness and sanitary order.

While various scholars have identified the importance of rendering certain spaces into zones of exclusion and of the physical delineation of a spatial periphery for the creation of geo-boundaries,[63] the Customs Quarantine Service and the new English System maintained very few permanently designated 'places' of isolation, inspection and exclusion at

British ports in the second half of the nineteenth century. In stark contrast, numerous other major shipping and immigrant destinations began and continued to invest heavily in such sites, most notably New York's Ellis Island, Sydney's North Head Quarantine Station, and Cape Town's Robben Island. Yet in Britain similar sites, where they continued to exist along its littoral, were falling into disrepair. Of the twenty-four stations that had been built around the British Isles (not including Ireland, which had an additional fifteen) during the seventeenth and eighteenth centuries, only five remained by 1870 when three more were closed. This left stations only at Liverpool and the Motherbank at Portsmouth, both of which were closed in the first half of the 1890s.[64] So, rather than constructing buildings as enduring symbols that 'operate[d] as thresholds that simultaneously embrace[d] and repulse[d]',[65] Britain relied more and more on temporary structures and the occasional use of floating hospitals for the reception of 'exotic' infections.

One of the first acts of the new Sanitary Authority in London was to acquire a hospital vessel for people who arrived with 'indigenous' disease, yet it also performed another significant symbolic function in announcing the presence of the new system. The old man-o'-war hulk *H.M.S. Rhin*, which had already been used by the Seamen's Hospital Society for the hospitalisation of cholera patients, was acquired with ease from the Admiralty. Prior to 1872, cases of cholera, arriving into London, were sent to the Hospital Ship *Dreadnought*[66] which was maintained by the Metropolitan Asylums Board.[67] However, with the new system in place the decision was made to abandon use of the *Dreadnought*, and acquire the *Rhin*.[68] Alterations were made within it, and a permanent mooring was established for it at Gravesend, alongside the Customs Authority, at the furthest point on the River Thames to which a ship could sail on any tide. Although not playing the same role in exhibiting a physical manifestation of the biological drawing and policing of the nation, as the imposing quarantine stations of New York or Sydney did for example, the *Rhin* clearly trumpeted the presence of the new Authority within the port. It heralded that the Customs Service was no longer the only official agency monitoring the health of arriving ships.

Months before the appointment of the first Medical Officer of Health for the Port of London, the *Rhin* was provided with two shipkeepers who were required to live on board the vessel with their wives, who acted as nurses and cleaners, and a medical officer, Dr Philip Whitcombe, was employed to run the six-bed hospital, care for the patients and oversee the maintenance of sanitary conditions on board the ship.

Whitcombe also filled the role of Port Medical Officer until the position was permanently filled by Harry Leach, who had previously worked at the Seaman's Hospital and as a medical advisor to the Board of Trade. The duties of the Port Medical Officer of Health, from the beginning, established the basic tenets of the English System, which worked on the sanitary and hygiene principles of disinfection, isolation and the sharing and collection of information.[69]

The duties of the Port Sanitary Officer, who was simultaneously appointed with Leach, related primarily to the inspection and maintenance of sanitary conditions on board vessels, such as ensuring the cleanliness of closets and latrines, that the crew and passenger quarters were sufficiently ventilated and that adequate cubic space was provided for each person on board. He was also responsible for executing any disinfection, cleansing and fumigation of vessels, goods and clothing, where instructed by the Medical Officer.[70] Both the duties of the Medical and Sanitary Officer were carried out in cooperation with the Quarantine Officers of the Customs Service, particularly in relation to cholera. Nevertheless, the position of the Port Sanitary Authorities as a separate and important organisation within the port was also guaranteed.

However, what most clearly demonstrated the establishment of the Port Sanitary Authorities as the new, additional and alternative system of disease prevention was the appointment of Whitcombe and the acquisition of the *Rhin* as a hospital to the Port Sanitary Authorities. While the Sanitary Committee acted with a degree of leisure in appointing a Port Medical Officer of Health and Sanitary Officer to oversee the health and sanitary condition of the port, the same leisure was not afforded in the establishment of the infectious disease hospital or to the appointment of its medical officer. The ship was a physical manifestation of the new authority in the port and demonstrated the Port Sanitary Authorities' appropriation of responsibility over the prevention of imported 'indigenous' disease. Located near the Customs Pier, the *Rhin* embodied the new Authorities as a counterpart to the role of the Customs Service and Privy Council in disease prevention at the port. The Port Sanitary Authorities cooperated with the other authorities still operating in the port such as the Customs Service and Seaman's Hospital Society, but the appointment of Whitcombe and the imposing presence of the new hospital ship immediately represented the authority of the new Port Sanitary system and the distinctive methods it would employ.

Over the following dozen years, the English System was further substantiated across port, maritime and urban spaces, in a number of additional laws. The authority of the Port Medical Officers in overseeing the sanitary standards and reception of infectious diseases in the port and riparian districts was finalised with the passing of the Public Health Act 1875.[71] Whereas the 1872 Act had put the Local Government Board in charge of assigning the powers and duties of the Port Sanitary Authorities, the 1875 Public Health Act granted the separate Port Authorities greater autonomy, although they ultimately still remained within the mandate of the Local Government Board.[72] A particularly important aspect of the 1875 Act was Section 130 which permitted the Local Government Board to alter or revoke any regulations in order for the Port Sanitary Authorities to prevent the spread of cholera.[73] The powers of the Port Sanitary Authorities were further consolidated with laws such as the Disease Prevention Act of 1883, which declared the Port of London Sanitary Authority to be an Urban Sanitary Authority, 'and giving the Local Government Board the power of assigning to them any such powers, rights, duties, capacities, liabilities and obligations as might appear to the Board to be required.'[74] The Public Health (Shipping) Act 1885 extended this and enabled the Port Medical Officers to act with more autonomy in executing sanitary procedures, for example cleansing or destroying items such as bedding on infected ships. It also enabled them to impose fines on shipping companies and captains who withheld information about possible infections.

With the death of Leach in 1879, a new Medical Officer of Health was needed for the Port of London. William Collingridge M.D., D.P.H., was a highly qualified physician who had been employed in private practice and in the military and saw the position of Medical Officer to the Port of London as a prestigious career move.[75] He remained in the post until replaced by Herbert Williams M.D., D.P.H., in 1901, who had been employed in the Port Sanitary Authorities as 'Medical Officer for Boarding purposes' since 1892. By the time Collingridge took up his post, the number of ships inspected in London had increased significantly from nearly 14,000 in 1874 to over 16,000 in 1880, and increasing to nearly 27,000 by 1883 (see Table 1.1).

However, as I explore in the next chapter, even as the English System was becoming deeply embedded in the working of ports around the country, international pressures on Britain to maintain and employ quarantine for cases of the traditionally quarantinable diseases as well as cholera continued into the final decade of the century. Meaning

Table 1.1 Return of vessels inspected, cleaned and fumigated and number of infectious disease cases dealt with – Port of London, 1873–93[76]

Year	Number of vessels inspected	Number of vessels cleaned	Number of vessels fumigated	Number of infectious disease cases dealt with
1873	1,999	338	9	83
1874	13,846	2,330	10	54
1875	14,847	1,788	5	120
1876	13,839	1,384	4	1
1877	14,310	754	10	3
1878	13,463	407	12	1
1879	14,804	516	6	–
1880	16,341	563	9	4
1881	22,315	428	30	28
1882	22,333	506	29	36
1883	26,833	1,102	22	19
1884	25,333	1,598	24	48
1885	24,327	1,819	33	32
1886	23,207	1,670	21	–
1887	21,855	1,744	23	110
1888	19,743	1,005	25	82
1889	19,396	606	19	36
1890	15,446	679	37	85
1891	15,341	402	27	76
1892	14,472	426	54	114
1893[a]	8,773	341	42	82
Total	362,823	20,416	451	1,057

[a] To end of July.

that, despite the progressive legislation that augmented the powers and position of the Port Sanitary Authorities in responding to all other infectious diseases, and its role in dealing with the few cases of cholera that had arrived since its inception, the English System remained in the shadow of quarantine legally and internationally.

Thus, when the *Rhin* began to show signs of serious deterioration and severe rotting, requiring a lengthy and expensive period of dry docking for the Admiralty to restore the ship to even a serviceable condition,[77] it was decided by the Port of London Sanitary Committee that both a more permanent and more suitable port isolation hospital was necessary in London. The Port Sanitary Committee argued that not only did the poor ventilation on board the *Rhin* 'retard recovery', but that the *Rhin* incurred an unnecessary expense which a land hospital would avoid.[78] For these reasons, and because it was important to demonstrate the permanence of the English System as a defining feature of British sanitary boundaries, the Corporation of London purchased a piece of land on which the hospital was built. The site lay at Denton, close to Gravesend and the old Customs House, and covered one and a half acres, with a river frontage of 100 feet. The new hospital, which contained an administration block, one ward for ten patients and a small single ward for 'better class patients or other specific purposes',[79] was formally opened on 17 April 1884. Unlike the massive quarantine and immigration stations built and maintained in New York or Sydney, for example, which were designed to accommodate the entire population of several shiploads of people at once, the Denton Hospital had the singular purpose of confining only those passengers or seamen who exhibited symptoms of disease. It was small and of limited use but it fulfilled the more potent symbolic purpose of establishing a permanent structure representative of the role of the Port Sanitary Authorities in defining a particular English System of disease control and making a particular 'British' sanitary zone.

Tensions and ambiguity

In late July 1873, a vessel called the *Iris* arrived into the Port of London full of European emigrants en route to New Zealand. It had two cases of cholera on board and was the first serious case of infectious disease since the establishment of the Port Sanitary Authorities. The ship had taken on board emigrants from Hamburg, Kiel and Copenhagen, and arrived in London with the appearance of a clean Bill of Health. However, six to eight hours after the emigrants reached their respective temporary lodgings in Whitechapel, two of the ship's passengers were attacked by the 'undoubted' symptoms of cholera. One of them, a child, died shortly thereafter, while the second, a man, was immediately isolated. The remaining 80 emigrants, with the assistance of the Whitehall and Whitechapel 'local authorities', were temporarily removed from their lodgings and taken to the *Rhin* for isolation and observation. The healthy were separated from the sick and were accommodated on board the S.S. *Osprey*, chartered by the emigration agency in charge of their passage to New Zealand. They remained on the *Osprey* until 17 August, when they were released back to the emigration agency. During this period, seven more emigrants developed symptoms of the disease and were admitted to the *Rhin*. The *Iris* had been placed in selected moorings off Deptford Creek when the infection was first detected. It was disinfected by the Port Sanitary Officer and released again within a few hours, causing 'a minimum of distraction to commercial interests'.[80]

In response to the *Iris* outbreak and the increasing likelihood that the cases were part of a larger epidemic, a temporary arrangement was put in place so that all vessels that arrived from 'suspected' ports were systematically examined at Gravesend.[81] However, despite the fact that various European vessels had rerouted to London to avoid Continental quarantines,[82] the only other cases of suspected cholera which were referred to the *Rhin* that summer were two seamen in mid-August and late September (only one of whom was recorded as suffering from cholera, while the other turned out to be merely a bad case of diarrhoea).

The significance of the *Iris* was that it was the first case of imported infectious disease dealt with by a Medical Officer of the Port of London. It marked a departure from procedures previously employed at the port and demonstrated a number of features particular to the English System. Most characteristic were the cooperative working of the Port Sanitary Authorities with local, inland, sanitary authorities, and the separation of the sick, as well as passengers believed to be at risk, from the ship on which they arrived. A peculiarity of the English System was that the health of the port was not separated from internal health – that is, the provision and administration of health and sanitary systems in localities outside port and riparian sanitary jurisdiction. The English System depended on communication and cooperation between port, riparian, urban and rural sanitary districts. Each separate branch of the sanitary system, although under local administration, operated within a national framework overseen by the Local Government Board. These relationships became increasingly complex but were based from this early stage on the idea of sanitary surveillance. This was a particularly important component of the English System whereby individual cases of disease could be recorded and monitored within and between localities, and the sanitary conditions of these localities were maintained at a high standard, so that disease could not spread.

Sanitary surveillance, which had extended out to the ports from urban and rural sanitary districts, turned around at the ports and looked back to local authorities to complete the system of maritime disease control. These local authorities set to the task of 'civilising' and containing the environment and populations within their districts, primarily within the poorest neighbourhoods. The homes and bodies of the poor were deemed to represent the greatest risk to ideals of cleanliness and order. According to Pamela Gilbert, 'The poor became not simply the victims of their own vice to be pitied or despised, but also enemies within. Once they had to be acknowledged as part of the social body, they became simultaneously more dangerous, more liable to be seen as foreign – wastes that had been expelled, yet reinvaded the body.'[83] The new science and social ideology of sanitation sought to control and enclose the spaces inhabited by the poor and the poor themselves, looking for 'filth' rather than contagion, and was committed to the reformative powers of enumeration, categorisation and surveillance.[84] It strove to identify, record and rectify – through fumigation, drainage or disinfection, for example – habitats of disorder and disease, making them more visible and manageable.[85] The English System brought the same principles and techniques to the control of disease that arrived into Britain's ports. Imported infections were not excluded from the lists, charts and tables that sought to impose order on the environmental and corporal well heads of disease. The ports, the ships within them and the people who arrived at them were all subject to the same mechanisms of control used in the poor neighbourhoods of Britain's towns and cities. It was this relationship between internal sanitary structures in local districts and the ports as places of arrival of vessels from foreign shores that distinguished the English System from other preventative systems, namely quarantine.

What was also particularly important in distinguishing the English System from quarantine was that the isolation of infectious cases, as well as suspected cases (where there had been some contact with the disease but no manifestation of it) did not occur on board the vessel upon which they arrived, nor were they detained together in a designated quarantine space. Infectious cases were removed as soon as possible to the isolation hospital maintained either by the port or riparian Authorities or local urban or rural Authorities. The sick were separated from the healthy, who were observed elsewhere. The vessel they arrived on was not detained for a period any longer than it took for it to be thoroughly disinfected, including, importantly, its bilge-water which was subsequently discarded. It was of great importance, as the case of the *Iris* demonstrates, that the presence of infection on board any vessel should cause only a modicum of delay to maritime traffic, and thus, as Leach had said, 'a minimum of distraction to commercial interests'. This also explains the importance attached to maintaining high levels of cooperation between the port and internal sanitary authorities. Usually, the infectious disease hospitals provided or used by the port Authorities accommodated only those who displayed symptoms of infectious disease. Yet, until the incubation period of a disease had elapsed,[86] other people on board a vessel could still be regarded as 'at risk'. The English System insisted on the separation of the sick from the healthy and rejected the notion of incarcerating the healthy during this period. It was generally only the sick who were kept and isolated by the Port Sanitary Authorities. Anyone who did not manifest symptoms indicating the presence of disease was free to disembark once details of his or her intended residence over the following days were recorded. These details were dispatched to the relevant local sanitary authorities who, for the known incubation period, observed the health of the passengers and crew of the vessel. The detention of the *Iris* passengers on board the *Osprey* for 18 days was thus not representative of the English System. Ordinarily, the health of uninfected passengers was monitored by the relevant local authorities and required only a minimum extension to the duties of the local medical and sanitary officers. This allowed the Port Sanitary Authorities to conduct their duties in such a way as to maintain the efficiency required at a busy and congested port such as London.

Nonetheless, from very early in the history of the Port Sanitary Authorities, the efficacy of the system was called into question. It was a problem that endured for twenty years and yet was at the heart of the Port Sanitary Authorities' role. Essentially, the predicament was that quarantine remained a legal obligation for the reception of vessels carrying plague or yellow fever and, as the quarantine law ambiguously stated, '*other infectious disease or distemper*[87] highly dangerous to the health of His Majesty's subjects'. This meant, in practice, that the Customs Service was legally obliged to approach the master of every ship that entered a British port and make enquiries into the health of all persons on board. As such, the first boarding authority on all ships was the Customs Service, operating under the Quarantine Law of 1825. The Port Medical Officer of Health did not board a vessel or examine the passengers or crew of a ship *unless* the Quarantine Medical Officer referred him to the ship. The Quarantine Officer questioned the master of the vessel and only sent for the Port Medical Officer if he discovered that an infectious disease, beyond the jurisdiction of the Quarantine Law, was present. It was only then that an employee of the Port Sanitary Authorities boarded a ship unless, as shall be demonstrated, particular circumstances prevailed. The Port Sanitary Authorities had jurisdiction only over those diseases deemed to be 'indigenous' to the British Isles. Diseases which were classified as 'exotic' were the responsibility of the Customs Service. The ports were therefore sited between two spatial domains – one which represented and sought to draw them within the domestic realm, and the other which embodied and reoriented the ports out into the broad 'foreign' space of the sea.

Furthermore, a Quarantine Medical Officer did not always board vessels with the Customs Boarding Officer. If a Customs Officer, while boarding a vessel alone, discovered a disease which was thought to be 'exotic', the Quarantine Medical Officer was brought to the ship to examine the case. In clearly 'indigenous' cases, the Port Medical Officer would be summoned. Sometimes the nature of the disease was unclear and it was only after the arrival of the Quarantine Medical Officer that the Port Medical Officer was summoned. The length of time this took naturally compounded the problems of having dual authority between the English System and quarantine.

The precise meaning and limits of the term 'other infectious disease or distemper' in the Quarantine Act was what proved most problematic. When the Act was passed in 1825 the only 'exotic' diseases at risk of being imported into Britain were plague and yellow fever. The first occurrence of cholera arrived some six years later, and subsequently it was unclear exactly how to deal with the disease. While the Quarantine Act remained the sole national system of port health, cholera mostly fell to the responsibility of the Customs Service – as it had during the epidemics from 1831–32 to 1866. However, responsibility and jurisdiction over cholera-infected ships became an increasingly complicated issue after the establishment of the Port Sanitary Authorities.

Reduced to its most simplistic terms, cholera could not be regarded as entirely within the jurisdiction of the Quarantine Service because it was not specifically named under the law, as plague and yellow fever were, and it was unclear whether it could be included under the provisions of *'other infectious disease or distemper'*. However, it was unquestionably identified as originating outside of Britain. Yet, if cholera did not fall strictly within the Quarantine Act, was it within the remit of the Sanitary Authorities? This was one of the predominant difficulties which the two authorities at the ports faced – who was responsible for dealing with the arrival of a cholera-infected vessel? Charles Follett, of His Majesty's Customs Solicitors' Department, when writing to the Privy Council later in the century, claimed that 'taking the [Quarantine] Act as it stands by itself ... that word [ie. "infectious"] has only, in my opinion, the limited meaning of quarantinable disease'[88] – by which he meant specifically plague and yellow fever. Yet, Customs impressed upon the Attorney General that the 'diseases intended to be touched by the Quarantine Acts' relate to 'plague and yellow fever because those are the diseases against which the Act was intended, but not meaning to exclude any other infectious exoteric [i.e. exotic] diseases, as for instance, Asiatic Cholera.'[89] This problem of jurisdiction remained until the repel of the Quarantine Act in 1896. Until then cholera-infected vessels generally required clearance from the Customs Service to enter a port and isolation and medical treatment of cholera cases was the responsibility of the Port Sanitary Authorities. However, this process altered at different times and sometimes in different ports, making it impossible to define a single procedure for cholera in the final quarter of the nineteenth century.

The problem of dual authority at the ports, shared between the Port Sanitary Authorities and Customs Service, was not confined to the ambiguity of jurisdiction over cholera. The identification, notification and inspection of other diseases also presented a quandary. While the Customs Service, for example, had the authority to detain vessels with an actual or suspected case of plague, yellow fever or cholera on board, it did not have the power to detain any other vessel. Even if, for example, a vessel was found by a Customs Boarding Officer to have a case of smallpox on board, the Officer could not legally order the detention of the vessel. This meant that the vessel could not be forced to remain at Gravesend by a Customs Officer, while the Port Medical Officer of Health was informed of the presence of the disease and was brought to the ship to undertake his own inspection. Subsequently, a vessel which carried a serious infection like smallpox could sail beyond Gravesend and into London, taking the disease with it.[90]

Members of the Port Sanitary Committee, in conversation with the Board of Trade, attempted to resolve this issue recommending an extension to the powers of the Quarantine Officers. They suggested, in late 1882, that the Quarantine Boarding Officers should have the power to detain vessels which carried *any* infectious illness for a 'reasonable period (say, six hours)', to allow time for communication with, and the arrival of, the Medical Officer.[91] The reply from Whitehall was negative, stating firstly that the laws of Quarantine were not cause for concern at the Customs Office, and secondly that it was not the place of the Sanitary Committee to 'take the initiative in proposing any alteration in the law..., that in the opinion of the Board of Customs any further restrictions than those at present in force would cause very serious inconveniences to the shipping interests'.[92] The Local Government Board supported this view and correspondingly sent a letter to the Committee. They agreed that any alteration to the law which increased the amount of time and number of vessels detained in the port would cause significant and unwanted 'inconveniences' to maritime traffic and attempted to redirect the problem to domestic 'coastal' vessels that were not examined by Customs Officers and were 'probably more likely' to spread infection than vessels from foreign ports.[93] Some serious issues were raised here in relation to the limitations of the Customs Service and the effectiveness of disease prevention under dual authority. However, because the suggested solutions would cause delays in maritime traffic the issue was dismissed.

The key problems in defining the respective roles of the Port Sanitary Authorities and the Customs Service continued to relate to both the ambiguous position of cholera and the notification of disease between authorities. Cholera perfectly characterised the lack of spatial definition represented at the ports. Neither the ports nor cholera could be neatly ordered within categories of 'foreign' or 'domestic', or 'exotic' or 'indigenous'. They were both seen as connected to the 'outside', while moving into and requiring responses from the 'inside'. Consequently, the effectiveness and role of the two authorities remained ill-defined well into the 1890s, for two reasons in particular. The first related to whether or not the failure of a master to report a case of 'indigenous' disease to a Customs Officer could result in prosecution. A master was required to give information about 'any sickness' which had occurred on board during the 'homeward' passage. Both of these terms were problematic. 'Any sickness' did not specify the important categorisation of 'indigenous' or 'exotic', and 'homeward passage' required an awkward valuation of sea space as either connected to 'home' or beyond the inclusive suggestion of 'homeward'. Masters could be prosecuted under the Quarantine Act if they failed to report an 'exotic' disease to the Customs Officer, in response to 'any sickness', but not if they withheld information about an 'indigenous' disease, and equally, they could be penalised for misinterpreting the limits of the 'homeward' passage.

The second reason related more specifically to cholera – to which authority should cholera be assigned? Although it was classified as an 'exotic' disease, cholera had not been specifically named under the Quarantine Act. Could the Act be applied to cholera-infected vessels; or should a Customs Officer refer cases of cholera to the Port Sanitary Authorities?

London's position as an imperial and maritime centre very quickly brought the first of these two problems to the attention of both authorities with the arrival into the East India Dock in May 1887 of the ship *Star of Austria* on its return from India. An inspector from the Port Sanitary Authorities examined the vessel having received information about a fatal case of remittent fever that had occurred on board during its voyage from the subcontinent. It had first stopped at Mauritius where the ship was placed in quarantine for three days and the quarters of the deceased crewmember were thoroughly cleaned and disinfected with sulphur. However, a case of cholera also occurred on the vessel while it was still in Calcutta. Before the vessel departed the man was removed to hospital and his belongings were destroyed. When the vessel arrived in London the master of the vessel omitted to give the Customs Boarding Officer information either about the case of remittent fever or, more importantly, the cholera:

> Although the vessel is not liable to Quarantine, the master would have to truthfully answer the preliminary <u>verbal</u> (sic) questions as to 'whence from', 'state of health', 'any infectious illness during voyage', and the like...
> If he had a case of cholera during the voyage or, as the words are, 'in the homeward passage' I should not hesitate to advise his prosecution, but his cholera case was all disposed of, bed and bedding and all, at Calcutta, with a clean Bill of Health there – while the case 'on the homeward passage' was only a feverish attack.[94]

It was argued that the master had not broken the law by either omitting the case of cholera, or by failing to inform the Customs Officer of the fatal case of fever which had occurred in the 'homeward passage'. The case of cholera occurred before the vessel undertook the voyage and thus the master was not required to declare it. It was also questionable whether the case of remittent fever was 'infectious'. Either way it remained uncertain whether the master had broken the law. If it was an infectious disease it was regarded as an 'esoteric or indigenous disease' and therefore not the responsibility of the Customs Service. As the Port Medical Officer for London, Collingridge, wrote in a report to Customs, the Quarantine Act 'only related to exoteric diseases and especially plague and yellow fever.'[95] If the case of remittent fever was not infectious, the master was not compelled to report it. Collingridge explained that there was neither any actual evidence of the infectiousness of the fever, nor was it considered to have posed any 'serious' threat to the public health.[96] However, the critical element here is that the *Star of Austria* illuminates the ambiguity surrounding the way disease and space were defined at the ports.

The conditions under which a master was required to declare an illness to the Customs Boarding Officer did not, as Collingridge observed, make things any easier:

> I know that the preliminary questions, often put in the wind and rain and with some difficulty are not put very formally, and the question, 'have you any <u>infectious</u> disease &c'. (sic) has grown into the question, 'any sickness', but the question is more or less a statutory one and the master is only bound to answer it truthfully according to its statutory limit.[97]

This 'statutory limit' was at the heart of the ambiguity. The law was particularly unclear regarding the absolute boundaries of these 'limits'. The problems of infectious disease categorisation and the boundaries of Port Sanitary and Customs Authorities, which the *Star of Austria* exposed, retreated from discussion for a few years, but came to the fore again in 1891 with the arrival of another ship, the *S.S. Memphis*. This vessel presented a similar array of problems to those encountered in 1887. In this case the diseases involved were the undeniably 'indigenous' enteric and typhoid fevers. Again the problem lay primarily in the question of whether or not a master was obliged to declare cases of 'indigenous' diseases, such as these, to the Quarantine Officer. In this case, it was unlikely that there could be a prosecution as it was determined that '"infectious", in deciding the question of Quarantine or not, means foreign and not indigenous disease, and ... that it may be doubted whether a master would be liable if his answer made no mention of an indigenous disease which happened to be, or have been on board'.[98]

As a result, it seemed feasible that unless changes were made in the law, or with regard to the Port Medical Officers of Health as a boarding authority, imported cases of 'indigenous' disease could pass through the 'first line of defence'. The problem was put to the Solicitor's Department of Her Majesty's Customs yet, but no clear evaluation or solution was forthcoming. No clarification was offered as to the position of the law on what diseases should be mentioned in reply to the quarantine questions, nor the responsibility under the law of the Customs Officers in determining the presence of disease, as the first boarding authority, for the officers of the Port Sanitary Authorities. The lawyer dealing with the case at the Solicitor's Department of Customs, Charles Follett, was unable to decipher what specifically was meant by 'other infectious disease or distemper highly dangerous to His Majesty's subjects', which was so crucial to achieving some clarity in the confusion surrounding the questions and the jurisdiction of both authorities. He asked the Attorney General what these diseases referred to in relation to the practical application of the Quarantine Act and the Public Health Act. According to the Privy Council, Follett explained, quarantinable diseases referred only to plague and yellow fever, although he maintained that these diseases were only the principal diseases against which the Act was aimed, and that the Act was 'not meant to exclude any other infectious, exoteric disease, as for instance, Asiatic Cholera'.[99] He suggested that the 'other infectious disease[s] or distemper[s]' could be a reference to 'infectious diseases placed under the charge of the Public Health Act'. This would solve the problem of what diseases masters were obliged to report. It would require 'an extension by Parliament of the meaning of the word "infectious" in the Quarantine Act' and would 'enlarge its meaning beyond what has, for many years been attached to it'.[100] However, the reply from the Royal Courts of Justice did little more than bring the problem almost full circle – returning it to the point from which it had begun.[101] And, for the time being, the issue was shelved.

A further problem associated with the quarantine questions was the necessity it placed on laymen to diagnose illness if there was no surgeon on board. The master of a vessel, with no medical knowledge, informed the Boarding Officer of any disease on board, but being a layman, incorrect statements were often made about the nature of the disease. This ignorance of medicine was also used as an excuse to conceal infectious diseases which, if discovered, might cause costly delays. However, such cases were almost impossible to prosecute as '...they could always plead, (if they had no surgeon on board) that they really didn't know, and believed the illness to be what they said'.[102]

Finally, the ambiguity, particularly in respect of cholera, was clearly captured in the utilisation of resources and facilities. As cholera was 'exotic', could quarantine hospitals be used by Medical Officers of Health for cholera cases; and what authority did relevant sections of the Public Health Acts have over Quarantine for the reception of this disease? In 1887, for example, the Privy Council on behalf of the Local Government Board appealed to the Law Officers' Department of the Royal Courts of Justice, requesting advice as to whether or not the two quarantine hulks, moored in the Motherbank, could be used 'for purposes other than strictly quarantine purposes, viz. for the reception of cholera patients.'[103] The reply from the Law Officers' Department was negative, suggesting only that either a new order be formed under the Public Health Act or the quarantine laws be reassessed with the purpose of broadening the scope of quarantinable diseases. As cholera was not strictly a 'quarantinable' disease, use of facilities maintained specifically for such diseases was not, under the law, allowed. Indeed they argued that any sharing of facilities would necessarily 'mix up' the functions of the different authorities and confuse things even more.[104] The letter demonstrates that not only were the powers of the sanitary authorities insufficient in allowing them to utilise quarantine facilities in the prevention of cholera, but also that cholera was considered sufficiently beyond the jurisdiction of the Quarantine Act for any of its facilities to be used in the prevention of the disease. Yet, although it may appear clear here that cholera was no longer felt to be the responsibility of the Customs Service, the example cited of the problems caused by the *Star of Austria* along with various others demonstrates that the nature and definition of cholera under the law remained ambiguous. It lay within an ill-defined 'in-between' space in the law and at the ports, neither 'indigenous' nor 'exotic' – 'inside' or 'outside'.

Conclusion

The Port Sanitary Authorities were established alongside an existing system of prevention at the ports which was very specifically focused in law and practice on one tightly defined category of disease, classified as 'exotic', pushed away from and kept outside of 'domestic' medical and preventative systems. Adding the sanitary system for the prevention of 'indigenous' disease at the ports meant, however, a necessary level of accommodation by the quarantine authorities which was difficult to achieve within the constraints of the law. Dual authority did not merely mean the addition of the Port Sanitary Authorities as separate entities within disease prevention but required mutual cooperation and compromise where there was an overlap in the function of the two authorities. As I have shown, the overlap in the boundaries and jurisdiction of the two authorities was an area which lacked legal or spatial clarity. Quarantine had clearly delineated internal and external spaces. The introduction of sanitary surveillance disordered the ports as places more clearly linked to the external than internal. It drew the border where imported diseases were prevented and controlled *in* from the ports, and widened the gap highlighted by the 1871 Sanitary Commission, creating a broader and more nebulous sanitary zone.

What was not ambiguous was that plague and yellow fever remained solely within the jurisdiction of the Quarantine Act. In June 1889 the last quarantine in Britain was imposed against the *S.S.Neva*, which arrived in Southampton from Brazil. On board was the body of one of three people who had died from an outbreak of yellow fever that had occurred on the homeward voyage. One patient was still in the acute phase of the disease. On arrival the Customs Officer and Quarantine Medical Officer came alongside, and learning of the cases ordered the vessel back out to sea to bury the body and then to return to the Motherbank in quarantine. Under orders from the Privy Council the infected man, with the ship's surgeon and two attendants, was removed to another vessel, the *Menelaus*, while the remaining passengers and crew were confined upon a third vessel, the *Edgar*. The *Neva* was disinfected with 'nitrous fumes' after which the crew was returned to it in order that it remained on its moorings. A special night watch was established to 'prevent intercommunication with those in quarantine', while precautions were made to ensure that personal contact was avoided when letters and provisions were delivered to each of the three vessels. Letters which were passed from the ships were fumigated before being despatched. The infected man – 'Andrews, the waiter' – died two days after the vessel arrived in Southampton on 13 June. No further cases were reported on either the *Neva* or *Edgar* and on 19 June the passengers and crew were released 'with great rejoicing, cheering, guns firing, and the like'. The surgeon and attendants were released from the *Menelaus* on 21 June.[105]

As the only example of its kind after the establishment of the Port Sanitary Authorities, this case not only demonstrates the procedures which were carried out on quarantined vessels in the late nineteenth century, but also shows that the practice had not entirely ceased to exist in British ports, as most of the existing scholarship claims.[106] Sanitation, as a preventative system and as a social and political mechanism, still had not penetrated the line quarantine drew around the British Isles in relation to the traditionally quarantinable diseases. Had more cases of yellow fever, or indeed plague, occurred prior to 1896 and after the establishment of the Port Sanitary Authorities, similar procedures would have been employed. Yellow fever and plague remained firmly under the Quarantine Act and, as the *Neva* demonstrated, the act was still enforced in the (rare) occurrence of these diseases during this period. However, Britain's response to cholera in the final quarter of the nineteenth century was what distinguished it from other quarantining nations.

Britain sought to define a space at its ports that signified a bio-political boundary. However, unlike the intransigent line drawn by quarantine policies in other parts of the world, the British geo-body was being defined as a more fluid construction. Port sanitation and sanitary surveillance were perfectly placed in the 'in-between' space of the littoral, bringing maritime disease control within the domestic public health infrastructure, yet keeping instances of infection at a safe distance. Rather than marking a geographical perimeter, the new English System established a sanitary zone that was more elastic and could be stretched or contracted to define different and changing constructions of 'inclusion' and 'exclusion'. Yet, even with such a system in place, the unpopular and incongruous principle and practice of quarantine continued, creating an unwieldy dual authority. The tension between the two functions of port health reflected friction between the two approaches to maritime disease control – one which was defined by the 'internal' (indigenous disease and domestic sanitary ideology) and the other by the 'external' ('exotic' diseases and exclusionary quarantines). It also illuminated the tensions implicit in the ports as the locus between 'foreign' and 'domestic' – politically as well as geographically. The following chapters will show how issues relating to port health had to navigate among the often conflicting demands of national and international interests, being pulled from both within and from outside. Lines of sovereignty became blurred, while perceptions of contagion were negotiated and renegotiated in the making of categories of disease and the 'diseased'.

Notes

1 Bashford, *Imperial Hygiene*, p. 123.
2 By the nineteenth century quarantine periods had been reduced from the medieval forty day period.

3 George Buchanan, *Fifteenth Annual Report of the LGB, 1885–6 –
Supplement Containing Reports and Papers on Cholera Submitted by the
Board's Medical Officer* (London: Eyre and Spottiswoode, 1886) [C. 4873],
p. ix.

4 For a fuller discussion of the various manifestations of 'Britishness' or
'British identity' see for example: Laurence Brockliss and David Eastwood
(eds), *A Union of Multiple Identities: The British Isles, c.1750–c.1850*
(Manchester: Manchester University Press, 1997); and Helen Brocklehurst
and Robert Phillips (eds), *History, Nationhood and the Question of Britain*
(London: Palgrave Macmillan, 2004).

5 John Seeley, *The Expansion of England: Two Courses of Lectures* (London:
Macmillan, 1914), p. 60. First published in 1883.

6 Duncan Bell, *The Idea of Greater Britain: Empire and the Future of World
Order, 1860–1900* (Princeton and Oxford: Princeton University Press,
2007), p. 7.

7 According to *Butterworth's Medical Dictionary* (London: Butterworth's,
1978) a 'Bill of Health' is 'An authenticated certificate concerning the
health of a ship's company and of the seaport, regarding infectious disease, which the master has to obtain before he may leave the port. The
certificate is "clean" when there is not any infectious disease at all,
"touched" or "suspected" when there are rumours of infection, and "foul"
when infection is certified'.

8 Michelle Allen, *Cleansing the City: Sanitary Geographies in Victorian
London* (Athens: Ohio University Press, 2008), p. 17.

9 William Collingridge, 'The Milroy Lectures – On Quarantine', Part 1,
BMJ, 13 March, 1897, 646–9, p. 646

10 *General Board of Health – Report on Quarantine*, 1849 [1070], p. 17.

11 Baldwin, *Contagion and the State*, p. 4.

12 Michael Brown, 'From Foetid Air to Filth: The Cultural Transformation of
British Epidemiological Thought, ca. 1780–1848,' *Bulletin of the History
of Medicine*, 82, 3 (2008), 515–44.

13 *Ibid.*

14 See chapter 2.

15 See John Booker, *Maritime Quarantine: The British Experience,
c.1650–1900* (Hampshire: Ashgate, 2007), pp. 279–83.

16 Evidence of William Matthias, Acting Superintendent of the Quarantine
at Milford, *Select Committee on Means of Improving and Maintaining
Foreign Trade – Second Report (Quarantine)* (1824) [417], p. 98

17 This process could take up to 15 days. Usually the contents of the hold
could only fit on deck in parts and thus airing needs to be completed in
stages. The first batch would be aired for six days and all subsequent
batches for only three days.

18 Matthias, *Select Committee (Quarantine)* (1824), pp. 99–100.

19 In 1798 Maclean was ordered to leave India for making an insinuation in an Indian newspaper against a magistrate. He left the East India Company after failing to make promotion and travelled for the Levant Company in 1815–17, *Concise DNB – Part One from the Beginnings to 1900* (Oxford: Oxford University Press, 1983), p. 820; see also, Brown, 'From Foetid Air'; Mark Harrison, *Public Health in British India: Anglo-Indian Preventive Medicine, 1859–1914* (Cambridge: Cambridge University Press, 1994), pp. 42–3; Pelling, *Cholera, Fever and English Medicine*, pp. 27–30; McDonald, 'The History of Quarantine', pp. 22–44; Erwin H. Ackerknecht, 'Anticontagionism between 1821 and 1867', *Bulletin of the History of Medicine*, 22 (1948), 562–93, pp. 582–5; and Roger Cooter, 'Anticontagionism and History's Medical Record', in P. Wright and A. Treacher, *The Problem of Medical Knowledge: Examining the Social Construction of Medicine* (Edinburgh: Edinburgh University Press, 1982), pp. 96–7.

20 Other texts include, Maclean, *Suggestions for the Prevention and Mitigation of Epidemic and Pestilential Diseases; Comprehending the Abolition of Quarantine and Lazarettos* (London, 1817).

21 Ackerknecht, 'Anticontagionism', p. 584.

22 Collingridge, 'On Quarantine' [Part1], p. 647, see also Catherine Kelly, '"Not from the College, But through the Public and the Legislature": Charles Maclean and the Relocation of Medical Debate in the Early Nineteenth Century,' *Bulletin of the History of Medicine*, 82, 3 (2008), 545–69.

23 *Select Committee (Quarantine)* (1824), p. 8.

24 McDonald, 'The History of Quarantine', p. 26.

25 Booker, *Maritime Quarantine*, p. 397.

26 *Ibid.*, p. 399.

27 Maclean died before the Bill was passed through to legislation.

28 Quarantine Act, 1825 (6 Geo. III c.78) II & III (my italics).

29 Richard Evans, *Death in Hamburg – Society and Politics in the Cholera Years* (Oxford: Clarendon Press, 1987), p. 226.

30 Baldwin, *Contagion and the State*, p. 101.

31 Longmate, *King Cholera*, pp. 24–5.

32 Evans, *Death in Hamburg*, p. 227.

33 McDonald, 'The History of Quarantine', p. 28.

34 Booker, *Maritime Quarantine*, p. 470.

35 Adrian Desmond, *The Politics of Evolution: Morphology, Medicine, and Reform in Radical London* (Chicago: University of Chicago Press, 1989), p. 16.

36 *London Medical Gazette*, 5 November 1831, p. 159.

37 Pelling, *Cholera, Fever and English Medicine*, p. 2.

38 *Report on the Mortality of Cholera in England, 1848–49* (London: HMSO, 1852), p. xlvii.

39 *Ibid.*, p. c.
40 Pelling, *Cholera, Fever and English Medicine*, p. 64.
41 *Report on Quarantine*, 1849, p. 17.
42 *Report on the Mortality of Cholera*, p. xlvii. See also, Christopher Hamlin, *Public Health and Social Justice in the Age of Chadwick: Britain, 1800–1854* (Cambridge: Cambridge University Press, 1998).
43 See chapter 2.
44 See Baldwin, *Contagion and the State*, pp. 147–9; Worboys, *Spreading Germs*, pp. 35–42 & 113–15; Pelling, *Cholera, Fever and English Medicine*, pp. 48–63; and Christopher Hamlin, *A Science of Impurity: Water Analysis in Nineteenth-Century Britain* (Bristol: Hilger, 1990), pp. 105–7.
45 *Report on the Mortality of Cholera*, p. c.
46 Christopher Hamlin, 'State Medicine in Great Britain', in Porter (ed.), *The History of Public Health*, pp. 132–64; and D, Porter, 'Public Health', in W.F. Bynum and Roy Porter (eds), *Companion Encyclopaedia of the History of Medicine*, vol. II (London: Routledge, 1993), 1231–61.
47 R. Thorne Thorne, 'On Sea-Borne Cholera: British Measures of Prevention v. European Measures of Restriction', *BMJ*, 13 August 1887, p. 340.
48 Hardy, 'Cholera', p. 255.
49 Collingridge, 'On Quarantine' [Part I], p. 648.
50 *Ibid.*
51 *Second Report of the Royal Sanitary Commission – Vol. I The Report* (London: HMSO, 1871) [C. 281], p. 51.
52 See chapter 2.
53 Evidence given by J.R. Slebbing [5911], *First Report of the Royal Sanitary Commission – With the Minutes of Evidence up to 5th August 1869* (London: HMSO, 1870) [C. 281], p. 330.
54 *Ibid.*
55 See for example, Brown, 'From Foetid Air'; John Pickstone, 'Dearth, Dirt and Fever Epidemics: Rewriting the History of British 'Public Health,' 1780–1850,' in Terence Ranger and Paul Slack (eds), *Epidemics and Ideas: Essays on the Historical Perception of Pestilence* (Cambridge: Cambridge University press, 1992), 125–48; and Christopher Hamlin, 'Edwin Chadwick, 'Mutton Medicine' and the Fever Question,' *Bulletin of the History of Medicine*, 70 (1996), 233–65.
56 *Second Report of the Royal Sanitary Commission*, p. 133.
57 *Ibid.*, p. 49.
58 Quarantine was actually still operational both in law and in practice, however rarely, when this quote was written in 1887.
59 Thorne Thorne, 'On Sea-Borne Cholera', p. 340.
60 For arrangements made at individual ports in anticipation of cholera in 1871 see, Appendix 47. 'First Report of the Local Government Board, 1871–2', *British Parliamentary Papers – House of Commons 1872*, 36296, vol. xxviii, pp. 334–6.

61 'Report by Dr. Blaxall on the Sanitary Survey of Port and Principal Riparian Sanitary Districts, 1885–6', *Fifteenth Annual Report of the LGB, 1885–6*, Appendix No. 8, p. 129.

62 Hardy, 'Public Health and the Expert', p. 135.

63 For example: Stern, 'Buildings, Boundaries and Blood'; Markel and Stern, 'Which Face? Whose Nation?'; Bashford, 'At the Border', 344–58; and Armstrong, 'Public Health Spaces' 393–410.

64 Booker, *Maritime Quarantine*, 574–7.

65 Stern, 'Buildings, Boundaries and Blood', p. 51.

66 See Cook, *From the Greenwich Hulks to Old St Pancras*, pp. 39–54; and Gordon C. Cook, *Disease in the Merchant Navy: A History of the Seamen's Hospital Society* (Oxford: Radcliffe Publishing, 2007).

67 'The Metropolitan Asylums Board had been set up in 1867 to provide and maintain hospitals and institutions in London for many branches of medicine, including infectious diseases', Cook, *From the Greenwich Hulks to Old St Pancras*, p. 51; see also, Gwendoline M. Ayers, *England's First State Hospitals and the Metropolitan Asylums Board, 1867–1930* (London: Wellcome Institute of the History of Medicine, 1971).

68 CLRO, *PSCP, 1872*. Letters from the Metropolitan Asylum District to the Port Sanitary Committee, Guildhall – 3 August 1872, and 26 August 1872.

69 CLRO, *Return of Corporation Appointments, 1879* (London: Charles Skipper & East Printers, 1879), p. 115.

70 *Ibid.*

71 Public Health Act, 1875 [38 & 39 VICT.], Section 287.

72 *Ibid.*, Sections 287–90.

73 *Ibid.*, Section 130.

74 William Collingridge, *The Duties of the Port Inspectors of Nuisances – For the Association of Public Sanitary Inspectors* (Whitechapel: Thos. Poulter & Sons, 1887), p. 29.

75 Collingridge was paid £500 per annum when appointed in 1880. His pay was increased to £700 per annum in 1884. When Williams was employed his salary began at £650 per annum. This was increased to £800 per annum in 1906. CLRO, *Return of Corporation Appointments, 1886* (London: Charles Skipper & East Printers, 1886); *Return of Corporation Appointments, 1908* (London: Charles Skipper & East Printers, 1908).

76 CLRO, *Royal Commission 1893 – City of London: Statement as to the Origin, Position, Powers, Duties, and Finance of the Corporation of London* (Guildhall, 1893), pp. 231–2.

77 CLRO, 'Hospital at Gravesend – Report to the Court of Common Council from the Port of London Sanitary Committee, 26 April 1883, *Printed Reports Index* [A/114F], p. 4.

78 *Ibid.*, pp. 5–6.

79 Patricia O'Driscoll, "'Against Infection and the Hand of War...' The Early years of the port health Service', *Port of London: Magazine of the port of London Authority*, 66 (1991), 65–9, p. 67.

80 CLRO, *PSCM*, vol. 1, 31 July 1873, Harry Leach, 'Special Report on Cholera'.

81 *Ibid.*

82 *Ibid.*, 2 Sept. 1873.

83 Pamela K. Gilbert, *Cholera and Nation: Doctoring the Social Body in Victorian England* (Albany: State University of New York Press, 2008), pp. 105–6.

84 *Ibid.*, 71.

85 Pamela K. Gilbert, *Mapping the Victorian Social Body* (Albany: State University of New York Press, 2004), p. 9.

86 Incubation periods for different diseases – particularly cholera – remained variable for much of the rest of the century.

87 My italics.

88 Nov. 1891, NA, PC8/447/67807.

89 Nov. 1891, NA, CUST46/95/25308.

90 See for example: 22 Sept. 1882, NA, MT10/375/H7298.

91 *Ibid.*

92 7 March 1883, NA, MT10/375/15710/83.

93 *Ibid.*

94 *Quarantine Regulations – Instructions to Service, 1887–1895*, NA, CUST46/95/12717.

95 *Ibid.*

96 *Ibid.*

97 *Ibid.*

98 NA, CUST46/95/11940.
    Part of this draft letter was crossed out but remains legible. It displays some disagreement about the infectious nature of some 'indigenous' disease:
    ...[it is understood] that Dr Collingridge is prepared to give an opinion that typhoid fever is infectious, although it is believed to be the opinion of certainly the great majority of medical men that this illness is not infectious, and that it prevails only epidemically in certain localities by each case having its origin in the same evil cause.

99 16 Nov. 1891, NA, CUST46/95/25308.

100 *Ibid.*

101 NA, CUST46/95/25309.

102 27 Dec. 1893, SRA CE60/1/89, p. 256.

103 NA, PC8/377/59669.

104 *Ibid.*

105 Blaxall, 'Report on the Steamship *NEVA* in Quarantine at the Motherbank, June 1889, on Account of Yellow Fever', *Nineteenth Annual Report of the LGB, 1889–90 – Supplement Containing the Report of the Medical Officer* (London: HMSO, 1890) [C. 6141-I], Appendix A No. 15, pp. 139–41.
106 For example: Hardy, 'Cholera'; MacDonald, 'The History of Quarantine'; Baldwin, *Contagion and the State*.

2

'Theoretical opinions...'

While the English System appeared to work well and to provide a satisfactory solution to the problem of imported infections in Britain, it remained shackled to the encumbrance of quarantine at home and abroad. Any approach to port disease control was intimately linked to international efforts to prevent imported epidemics; this was particularly so in relation to the problem of cholera, which, it was clear by mid-century, was not going away. Cholera crossed, permeated and dissolved national borders and spaces and severely undermined growing imperial networks. New technologies that permitted unimaginably rapid global travel and connections brought with them an increased threat and sense of vulnerability to the most feared diseases, plague, yellow fever and cholera. However, the systems and responses put in place around the world to arrest the spread of these infections were inconsistent and obstructive, contradictiously undermining the 'new velocity of transport' and interfering with the ever growing profits it generated.[1] Most nations looked to quarantine to defend their cities and populations, but the qualifying factors, duration and conditions of these quarantines often seemed arbitrary and certainly unsystematic. The international problem of epidemic disease, in particular cholera, while dealt with locally or nationally, and differing from place to place, was becoming increasingly untenable. Thus, in 1851, in the context of a proliferation of international meetings, the first International Sanitary Conference was held in Paris with the aim of standardising the control of disease between regions and across borders.

Disease prevention in British ports was, with the dual authority, 'two-pronged' between the foundation of the English System in 1872 and the abolition of quarantine in 1896.[2] What most scholarship which has sought to address this period has failed to take into consideration in its assessments of port prophylaxis was the international negotiations and pressures which were exerted on Britain with regard to quarantine. Although Britain had established a unique system of sanitary control for infectious disease which enabled the country to be less reliant on quarantine as the first and only line of defence, British preventative strategies could not be separated from contemporary quarantine policies, practices and theories which existed beyond British shores. So, even though a system was being created and increasingly defined by 'English' sanitary practice, quarantine maintained a significant hold over Britain's relationship with other nations with regard to disease control in the international arena.

The way that Britain dealt with the arrival of vessels into its own domestic ports carrying infectious disease was greatly determined by the external pressures put on it by primarily European powers and large imperial shipping and trading companies. I have stressed that one of the key, if not most important, factors which influenced British opposition to quarantine was its effect on trade and commerce. The enormous expense caused by quarantine, the apparent futility of the system as an effective method of disease control and the restrictive national boundaries which quarantine implied were weighty reasons for Britain to abolish the use and legal obligation of the practice particularly from the 1870s, when an apparently superior and eminently more suitable method of prevention had been established. Yet, external pressures to maintain quarantine were such that the difficulties of dual authority continued in the ports into the middle of the 1890s. Previous scholarship, without extending its analysis beyond the bounds of Britain and subsequently overlooking the importance of international opinion and other external pressures, has been unable to account for the continued presence of the Customs Service in port prophylaxis into the 1890s and has subsequently ignored the complexities and ambiguities which the continued dual authority entailed.

The contagion/anti-contagion debate

The political importance of quarantine in international affairs is not a new area of enquiry. Scholars as far back as Erwin Ackerknecht in 1948 have explored the relationship between disease control and politics, examining their connections and implications for science and aetiology, geography and economic systems.[3]

In his seminal essay, widely understood to be one of the 'best known' and 'most influential' articles in the modern history of medicine, Ackerknecht initiated several decades of discussion when he asserted that there was a direct link between the political systems and disease control practices of states, and that this relationship was bound together with correlating notions of disease causation.[4] While contested by a number of scholars, the connections established by Ackerknecht under-lie all subsequent analyses of international quarantine and attempts to achieve cooperation and standardisation of practices. His thesis cen-tred on the assertion that anti-contagionism – theories of disease trans-mission based on miasma, environment and localism – was endowed with scientific respectability and reached a crescendo up to the middle of the nineteenth century but was beginning to decline from the 1850s in favour of contagionism and the eventual ascendance of germ theory. What motivated these trends, he argued, was not forces intrinsic to medicine itself but the powerful personal and collective political and socio-economic perspectives of physicians and policy makers. Each of the theories contained both sufficient uncertainty and plausibility to allow physicians to judge them also by their practical outcomes, mean-ing that prevailing political ideology became intrinsic to medical theo-ries of disease transmission. As Ackerknecht explained:

> Intellectually and rationally the two theories balanced each other too evenly. Under such conditions the accident of personal experience and temperament, and especially economic outlook and political loy-alties will determine the decision. These, being liberal and bourgeois in the majority of the physicians of the time brought about the victory of anticontagionism. *It is typical that the ascendancy of anticonta-gionism coincides with the rise of liberalism, its decline with the vic-tory of the reaction.*[5]

Contagionism was the underlying principle of quarantine and cor-dons sanitaire, which had come to be characterised by heavy-handed restrictions and intrusion equal to that of the authoritarian regimes that imposed them. Ackerknecht was unequivocal in his drawing of the relationship between quarantine and contagionism, stating that 'the whole discussion [of contagionists] was thus never a discussion on contagion alone, but *always on contagion and quarantines*.'[6] Anti-contagionism on the other hand was, as the name implies, defined not only by its belief in the environmental origin of disease but also by its opposition to the medical and political doctrine of contagion. It focussed on both local sanitary improvement in the form of sewerage disposal, street cleaning, housing regulations and so on, as well as that other fundamental aspect of the sanitary movement, social reform. Anti-contagionists were, in their opposition to quarantine and support of the sanitary movement therefore, as Ackerknecht argued, 'reformers, fighting for the freedom of the individual and commerce against the shackles of despotism and reaction'.[7]

Subsequent studies, particularly those which have analysed national and international disease control measures, have criticised the broad brush strokes applied by Ackerknecht, showing through more detailed work, that the dichotomous relationships he drew are too insufficient to account for all the contingencies in theory and practice.[8] The contagion/anti-contagion binary does not allow for the wide array of theories that rose, fell and were sustained throughout the period – even though Ackerknecht discussed a middle group which he called 'contingent contagionists' – or account for the great many physicians who moved in and between or combined ideas of contagion and environment at different times and in different contexts. Peter Baldwin has challenged Ackerknecht's neat summation of prophylaxis and politics, stating rather that the geographical proximity of a State to the source of infectious disease was the key determinate in the way it responded to epidemics. Thus the simple equation of liberal or authoritarian could be exchanged for what Baldwin calls 'geoepidemiology' in explaining the use of either quarantines or sanitary measures. He boldly concludes that not only did geoepidemiology shape prophylaxis but it also formed 'the very political traditions of these nations'.[9] His argument is compelling but, like with all such formulas, is too neat to allow for variations over time and in changing circumstances.

Ultimately, despite the challenges to Ackerknecht's thesis, the framework for analysis it offers remains valuable. Indeed, even beyond the chronological scope of his essay, the sources appear to support the idea that political expedients were if not determining then certainly influential in the policies, practices and science of port prophylaxis. As we shall see, while there was a great variety of views amongst physicians about the aetiology of cholera, in particular, in the later part of the nineteenth century, a relatively consistent politicised position was maintained in Britain in relation to theories of epidemic transmission in port and maritime disease control. These did not always conform to the convenient binary of contagion versus anti-contagion but the two sets of theories, rhetorically at least, underlay the politically oppositional practices of quarantine and sanitation.

By the last quarter of the century the terms contagion and anti-contagion had changed somewhat in meaning and connotation from the early part of the century. Being 'contagionist' implied a belief in the theory of disease aetiology which held that a specific disease entity, or 'germ', independent of locality, was the causative agent of disease, and that this organism could pass from one person to another either though exhalations or excreta.[10] Not all organisms had been specifically identified by the early 1880s, yet contagionists accepted their role in the transmission of disease.[11] 'Anti-contagionists', no longer the 'miasmatists' of earlier decades, were called 'non-contagionists' by contemporaries and occupied more of the 'middle-ground' of Ackerknecht's 'contingent contagionists'. They generally did not dispute the *possibility* of an infective agent, but required for a disease to take hold the predisposing factors of an individual's general 'sickly' constitution and, most importantly, an environment of filth, bad ventilation, general uncleanliness, and for some, meteorological and climatic conditions. The dominance of this 'middle ground' in Britain is evident throughout the medical discourse of public health. In 1885, for example, two years after Robert Koch identified cholera's causative bacteria, George Buchanan, Chief Medical Officer of the Local Government Board, wrote in his Annual Report that 'when a case of cholera is imported into any place, the disease is not likely to spread, unless in proportion as it finds, locally open to it, certain facilities for spreading by *indirect infection*'.[12] Even well into the 'bacteriological age' divisions still remained between the two aetiological camps primarily, as we shall see, in connection with their implications for port and maritime prophylaxis. So, although through his acknowledgement of the 'contingent contagionists' Ackerknecht accepted a wider interpretation of medical theories than the simple dichotomy of contagion and anti-contagion, his argument, and mine, is that the polarisation lay not in medical theory but in the practical application of prophylaxis at the ports – quarantine or sanitary inspection.[13]

However, even this dichotomy may be challenged. Michael Worboys argues that the practical applications of disease theories in preventative public health were divided into 'inclusive' and 'exclusive' programmes. 'Inclusive' practices focused entirely on prevention through environmental improvements and adhered to anti-contagionist, miasmatic theories of disease. 'Exclusionary' methods were any which aimed to prevent the transmission of disease from person to person, and used, for example, disinfection or isolation.[14] The latter focused on individuals rather than the environment in preventing disease. As Worboys points out, historians generally place the transition of public health from environmentally centred policies to those focused more on individuals to around the late 1880s and 1890s. Yet he argues that increasing emphasis on the 'exclusive' methods of isolation, notification and disinfection through the 1870s, 'shows that person-centred approaches were ... used much earlier'.[15] Indeed, the duties assigned to Leach and his sanitary officers in London at the inception of the Port Sanitary Authority in 1873 were particularly focused on the use of disinfection and isolation of the sick. This example both further enforces Worboys's claim for an earlier introduction of these practices and also demonstrates that 'exclusion' was integral to the English System through its incorporation of practices aimed at preventing person-to-person infection. Yet, the English System also relied heavily upon the 'inclusionary' preventive methods of continuing and maintaining environmental improvements in the port, in internal sanitary districts and aboard vessels. The simple dichotomy of sanitary inspection versus quarantine at the ports as a divide between environmental sanitary methods and exclusionary quarantines does not, then, work in Worboys's model. The English System therefore sits as a practical application of the same 'middle-ground' occupied by contingent- (or non-)contagionist theories. Nevertheless, although neither the medical theoretical nor practical prevention of infectious diseases can be easily dichotomised, for the purpose of both my argument and the argument of those involved in the nineteenth century, the terms of discussion are polarised.

There were shifts within aetiological thinking in the 1880s and 1890s in response to developments in bacteriology and laboratory medicine, yet even so, the politically important implications of infectious disease transmission at the ports maintained notions of non-contagionism among physicians involved in port prophylaxis well into the so-called 'bacteriological era'. This oriented port health more toward the theories of disease transmission maintained in India than those which were being developed within Britain.[16] This was most clearly articulated at the International Sanitary Conferences of the second half of the nineteenth century, where it was unambiguously shown that the theories promoted by the British and Colonial Indian delegates were those which unequivocally supported their economic and political interests in maritime trade and trade routes. Despite various developments in understandings of infectious disease aetiology made during the second half of the century, Britain's political and medical position at the conferences was almost entirely without modification between the first conference held in 1851 and those held in the late 1880s and early 1890s. The non-contagious nature of cholera, and to a lesser extent plague and yellow fever, was the basis of Britain's objection to quarantine in both the domestic and international sphere. Non-contagious disease theories, and those which were contingent on location, provided medical justification for opposing maritime quarantines and were maintained almost unwaveringly by British delegates over five decades of international conferences, despite the often overwhelming resistance of other representative States.

Internationalising cholera

The International Sanitary Conferences of the nineteenth century are often seen, teleologically, to be precursors to the international cooperation embodied in the World Health Organisation, setting the stage for cross-cultural discussion about the health of populations and the prevention of disease. Indeed, they originated in a post-Congress of Vienna milieu of growing internationalism and a proliferation of scientific, diplomatic and cultural conferences and congresses seeking to set standards and share new knowledge and technology. Thus the first International Sanitary Conference convened in Paris in 1851 was held in the same year as the Great Exhibition at the Crystal Palace and within the context of international agreements regarding, among many other things, maritime traffic, telegraphic communication, patents and copyright, and the standardisation of weights and measures. While called 'international' however, the sanitary conferences were predominantly attended by European delegates and were primarily concerned with preventing the introduction of plague, yellow fever and cholera into Europe (Table 2.1). The way different European States responded to extra-European disease threats depended on a combination of geography, political culture and commercial and imperial interests which sometimes changed along with shifting relationships among and between the different States. Britain, however and as I have already indicated, maintained an almost uniquely consistent stance at the conferences, and it is its contribution to the meetings that will be my focus for the remainder of this chapter, particularly the way the meetings and their content were shown to have direct bearing on the development of policy and practice in Britain's domestic ports.

With efforts at bringing together an international meeting having been shelved during the revolutions of 1848, the first International Sanitary Conference was initiated by France and attended by representatives of twelve European States (including Turkey).[17] Obstructive quarantines in the Mediterranean had been frustrating France as it increased its trading activities in North Africa, a dissatisfaction that was shared by other nations including Britain and Austria.[18] However, after a few abortive attempts by the British and French governments in the 1830s and 1840s, in the wake of Europe's first encounter with epidemic cholera, to bring together an international conference on quarantine, the first conference was opened on 23 July 1851. Its central agenda was to fix a minimum requirement for maritime quarantine in order, as the President of the Conference explained in his opening speech, to render 'important services to the trade and shipping of the Mediterranean, while at the same time safeguarding the public health'.[19]

The conference, which was attended by a diplomatic and medical representative from each of the represented States, lasted six months and consisted of forty-eight plenary sessions and numerous committee meetings. By the close of proceedings on 19 January 1852, a convention had been produced in draft form and was signed by all twenty-four delegates (two from each country). However, only three of the twelve States signed the final draft of the convention and of these only Sardinia ratified the agreement.[20] Part of the problem was that voting was undertaken by individual representatives rather than by country. Fundamental difficulties resulted from trying to reconcile the opinions, not only of the different governments, but of the diplomatic representatives and the physicians who often disagreed about underlying issues relating to the regulation of shipping during epidemics.[21]

At the heart of the conference's discussions was whether cholera was 'epidemic', 'infectious' or 'contagious' despite it having been agreed from the outset that 'scientific theories should not be discussed but practical solutions sought'.[22] Loosely defined in contemporary understanding of the terms, 'epidemic' disease was determined by particular meteorological conditions or conditions of the soil, striking large numbers of people but not transmitted from person to person. 'Infectious' disease was transmitted from one person to another through exhaled poisons or miasma; while 'contagious' disease was transmitted by 'morbid matter' from person to person directly or indirectly, or through fomites, either as a 'living' entity or not.[23] In an attempt to steer the deliberations away from cholera and toward yellow fever and plague, the Austrian medical delegate, G.M. Ménis, declared that cholera was a 'purely epidemic disease' and therefore did not need to be discussed in relation to quarantine.[24] Britain and France keenly supported this notion; indeed Britain firmly maintained the position throughout the proceedings that quarantine, for any of the three disease categories, was unnecessary. Only two years prior to the conference, Britain's medical delegate, John Sutherland, a medical inspector at the General Board of Health, had contributed to the *Report to the General Board of Health on the Epidemic of Cholera of 1848 and 1849.*[25] The Board, the hard won creation of Edwin Chadwick and other sanitarians, was rooted in theories of localised disease causation and the parallel predisposing causes of squalid living conditions, filth and overcrowding. It, and the report written by Sutherland, dismissed John Snow's conclusions about water transmission following his study of the Broad Street pump, and instead concluded that cholera resulted from foul air and miasmas which were particularly harmful among people whose constitutions predisposed them to cholera through living in filth and lacking moral rectitude.[26] Sutherland brought these ideas and the support of the Board to the conference, neglecting to mention Snow's report and encouraging proposals that discouraged the use of quarantine. In England it was widely believed, wrote Britain's diplomatic representative to the conference, Anthony Perrier, that 'contagion is not a fact, but an hypothesis invented to explain a number of facts that, without this hypothesis, would be inexplicable'.[27]

France adopted a position more in favour of compromise, while the delegates of the remaining countries argued for a greater or lesser degree of some form of quarantine, depending very much on whether they were a medical or diplomatic representative. However, regardless of whether or not the medical delegates were able to reach some sort of agreement on the mode of cholera or plague transmission, each of the diplomatic representatives had been sent with the particular political and commercial agendas of their respective governments concerning quarantine. This neither necessarily accorded with current medical theories nor the opinion of the medical representative. Thus, with no agreement reached after six months of discussion either on modes of transmission or the duration or conditions of quarantine, the conference ended without resolution. None of the regulations drawn up in the convention were either ratified, except by Sardinia, or otherwise adhered to, and so, despite the fact that the conference set a precedent for further international discussion and cooperation, it was completely unsuccessful in achieving any of its initial aims. As the President of the Epidemiological Society of London, Professor J.L. Notter, reminisced in an address to the Society in 1898, 'for all practical purposes the results of this conference were unsatisfactory; there was little unity of opinion, and no system of International control was possible under the circumstances'.[28]

The second conference, held again in Paris eight years later, was an endeavour to salvage some of the collaborative work of 1851. Attempting to simplify the text and the proceedings of the second conference, and in order to try and reach a more mutually agreeable and manageable convention, only diplomatic representatives were invited to attend the conference. Surprisingly, this did not prevent fierce debates dividing the contagionist and anti-contagionist camps, although the majority of discussion during the five months of the conference contained minimal medical content. The conference produced a draft convention, which sought to reconcile the apparent impasse, but again it was not signed or ratified and each State resumed individualised protection at their ports and frontiers, meaning that the myriad of preventive systems continued to complicate maritime traffic.

The next two conferences held in Constantinople in 1866 and Vienna in 1874 followed a similar pattern to the first and second conferences. That is, the Vienna conference was essentially a review and reworking of the resolutions of the Constantinople conference. Both conferences were devoted entirely to the examination of cholera and the best means of preventing its spread. This meant that they were more medically based than the 1859 conference and that current aetiological and epidemiological theories of the disease were more central to the discussion.

The Constantinople conference was held toward the end of one of Europe's worst encounters with epidemic cholera in 1865–66. For the first time the disease had arrived in Europe by sea from Egypt. Previous epidemics had arrived largely overland from Eastern Europe, brought west from India to the Middle East by Haj pilgrims. From 1858, however, the new Alexandria-Cairo-Suez railway line combined with sea transport to open up faster and more direct connections to pilgrimage sites in the Hijaz, and in 1865 a particularly virulent outbreak of cholera combined with the vastly more busy *Hadj al-Jum'a* which put many more pilgrims on the move from India as well as other places.[29] Consequently, it was widely understood at the conference that Muslim pilgrims were the chief conduits of the disease into Europe and that disease control in Iran, Turkey, Russia and Egypt was key to the safety of Western Europeans. Responding to these assumptions, amongst the most significant resolutions of the third conference was the almost unanimous conclusion that cholera had originated in India, that humans were the principal agent in the transmission of the disease and that, despite the fact that previous epidemics had almost certainly arrived in Western Europe via land routes, maritime communications were the foremost means of disseminating the disease, followed by railway contact.[30] The only abstention from this conclusion came from Dr. E. Goodeve, one of the British delegates. The Government of India had not been permitted to send a representative to the conference but 'found a champion' in Goodeve, who had held a senior position at Calcutta Medical College.[31] Not surprisingly, he and the other British delegate were resistant to the implication of the resolution that cholera had been brought to Europe through British imperial enterprise. The suggestion that, as India was the recognised origin of cholera, an international medical team should be sent there to investigate the disease also met with British objections. Yet, the British delegates did concede that there was some British responsibility toward arresting the further spread of the disease, and examples of sanitary work already underway in the ports of Bombay, Calcutta and Madras were provided.[32]

Greatly significant to the discussion of cholera at both the third and fourth conferences were the aetiological theories of Max von Pettenkofer (1818–1901). Allowing for the possibility that the 'excrementitious matters' expelled from the bodies of cholera sufferers played a part in the transmission of the disease, Pettenkofer did not alienate traditional contagionists. However, his theory insisted that certain predisposing environments and constitutions were necessary for an epidemic to occur. Thus, medically and politically divergent delegates at the 1866 conference unanimously agreed that:

> the hygienic and other conditions which in general predispose a population to contract cholera, and, consequently, favor the intensity of epidemics, are: misery, with all its consequences, the accumulation of individuals, impaired health, the warm season, want of ventilation, and exhalations from a porous soil impregnated with organic matters, particularly if these matters come from cholera dejections.[33]

What was most appealing about Pettenkofer's theory was that it stood midway between a contagionist and anti-contagionist understanding of disease transmission. He claimed that in order for cholera to develop, both the importation of the 'germ' into a locality and particular local meteorological and soil conditions and constitution were required. He accepted that disease could be transmitted from one locality to another, but not from one person to another. However, his theories accommodated in different ways both the medical and political rationalisations for quarantine and sanitation, and so were a useful basis for discussion among otherwise divided delegates. It was, thus, with much of his influence that the conference concluded that while a quarantine of up to ten days would be necessary for vessels with a foul Bill of Health, cordons sanitaires were pointless in highly populated, filthy urban areas (which might be said to have included many of the world's major ports) and that improving the sanitary conditions – provision of clean water and preservation of the purity of the air – of ports and towns was an important determinant in the prevention of epidemic cholera.

In the eight intervening years between the third (1866) and fourth (1874) conferences, Pettenkofer further clarified his theory of the aetiology of cholera. According to his theory, the interaction of three factors was the cause of epidemic cholera.[34] Each of these factors – the germ (x), the local and seasonal conditions (y) and an individual's predisposition (z) – were all required in the development of the disease – which occurred as a process of 'fermentation' – but the most important, according to Pettenkofer, was the environment, particularly the condition of the soil. Theoretically, therefore, cholera could be imported but only if the seasonal conditions and soil, and the constitution of the local population, were such that the disease could 'take hold'. The germ itself, Pettenkofer argued, was incapable of causing cholera.[35] However, although Pettenkofer had many followers within Britain at this time, theories more weighted toward environmental factors still carried great favour. (John Simon, Medical Officer of Health to the Privy Council, for example, attributed the propagation of cholera, and other 'infectious' diseases, to 'filth' of all varieties.)[36] However, Pettenkofer's abstention, as one of the two German delegates at the Fourth International Sanitary Conference in 1874, from the same conclusion made at the third conference that cholera was always imported to Europe from India, won him much support in Britain and India. The political expediency of his theory meant that Britain and Colonial India adopted it at this conference and those which followed, providing the necessary scientific rationale and support of British maritime trade interests to and from India. As Mark Harrison has argued in relation to the Government of India's use of Pettenkofer's scientific expertise, his 'aetiological positions did not so much determine, as provide a justification for, existing sanitary policies'.[37] Pettenkofer argued strongly that local conditions were essential to the propagation of cholera and, such was the weight of his argument in Vienna in 1874 that the representatives of this largely contagionist conference voted unanimously on a resolution which took some account of Pettenkofer's theories:

> The Conference accepts the transmissibility of cholera by man coming from an infected environment; it considers man as able to be the specific cause only outside the influence of the infected locality; further, it regards him as the propagator of cholera when he comes from a place where the germ of the disease already exists.[38]

However, yet again there was no ratified convention signed at the end of the proceedings, despite very strong moves having been made toward establishing a permanent International Sanitary Commission in Vienna with the remit of studying epidemic diseases. What did come out of the 1874 conference, however, was a unanimous resolution that, as no mutually acceptable agreement on maritime quarantine could be reached, each country would have the right to choose between *either* a system of quarantine or sanitary medical inspection. This was of great significance to Britain which had only just established the Port Sanitary Authority, based on a system of sanitary surveillance. Richard Thorne Thorne (then Deputy Chief Medical Officer to the Local Government Board),[39] who had been Britain's medical delegate, reminisced about the importance of this resolution after he participated in the Sixth Conference held in 1885, where the decisions had been 'of a retrograde character' compared with the conference of 1874. He explained, 'I undertook to give ... some notion of the sanitary work that had been affected in this country since the system of medical inspection had, with the approval of the Vienna Conference in 1874, superseded all attempts at quarantine both on our shores and inland'.[40] While still largely in favour of cordons, the 1874 conference allowed sufficient space for Britain to begin pursuing an alternative preventive system, even though quarantines might remain necessary 'outside' of Europe.

The next conference differed in character and content from those of the previous decades. Seven years after Constantinople, the fifth conference was convened in Washington, marking a departure from the Eurocentricity of preceding conferences. Although the United States had been invited to the previous two conferences, they had declined to attend. This time they hosted the conference and it was attended not only by European States, together with Turkey and Egypt, but also several North and South American nations as well as China and Japan, making it one of the most internationally representative conferences of the nineteenth century. Although cholera and yellow fever had attacked the Americas during the century, issues regarding the quarantining of these diseases had been discussed at the first four conferences only with reference to Europe, the Middle-East (particularly in relation to Muslim pilgrimages) and the Indian subcontinent. However, with continuing trade and the intensification of migration across the Atlantic, the threat of these diseases taking hold with greater frequency in both hemispheres prompted the United States to enter into international discussions about quarantine procedures. A joint resolution of the Senate and the House of Representatives agreed upon America's need to join an international sanitary agreement and submitted that America should host the fifth conference. Providing an axis for discussion at the conference were the two key issues:

> The establishment of a reliable and satisfactory international system of notification as to the existence of contagious and infectious diseases, more especially cholera and yellow fever.
> The establishment of a uniform and satisfactory system of Bills of Health, the statements in which shall be trustworthy as to the sanitary condition of the port of departure and as to the condition of the vessel at the time of sailing.[41]

Further to the United States' desire to include a greater representation of the world's major trade routes in the pursuit of internationally agreed quarantine procedures, and to examine the possibility of reaching international agreement on the above, the meeting was summoned to attend to matters of a more domestic nature. Norman Howard-Jones, whose 1974 series of articles is still the most thorough, has asserted that 'the sole objective of the USA in convening this conference was to obtain international assent to a piece of domestic legislation that would otherwise be unenforceable'.[42] The National Board of Health Act was passed in 1879 to protect against 'the introduction of contagious or infectious diseases into the United States', and required specifically that 'all merchant ships and vessels sailing from a foreign port where contagious or infectious disease exists, for any port in the United States, must obtain from the consul ... at the port of departure ... a Bill of Health'.[43] The provisions of the Act were such that all ships departing from a foreign port bound for America were required to be in possession of a Bill of Health and 'sanitary history' endorsed by a United States Consular Official working in that foreign country. This required the Consular Official, as well as the Port Officials of the country of departure, to inspect the ship. 'It is hardly surprising', Howard-Jones points out, 'that difficulties arose in the enforcement of such a law, and it was evidently the realisation on the part of Congress that the Act must necessarily remain a dead letter unless other nations could be persuaded to agree to it that led to the idea of an international conference'.[44] This motive for convening the conference was never disguised by the United States. In fact, the necessity for obtaining international cooperation in order to achieve the aims of a piece of domestic legislation was announced in the conference's opening speech.[45]

The proposal was opposed by a majority of representative countries for numerous reasons including the belief, put forward by Italy and Spain, that a medical inspection and certificate of health provided by officials of the port of departure should be sufficient proof in assuring the absence of disease and that the request for independent examination suggested otherwise. Britain raised the issue of sovereignty and rejected the proposal on the grounds that it would be both impractical and an infringement of sovereign power. Ultimately, the United States was unsuccessful in attaining the international assent and cooperation required to fulfil the objectives of the Act.[46] The conference was, as a result, more concerned with managerial and administrative matters than with scientific concerns or the latest innovations in infectious disease prevention, although there was some discussion about the aetiology of yellow fever.

Rome, 1885

It was, in part, due to the lack of scientific discussion at the Washington conference that only four years later the next conference was held again in Europe, this time in Rome. Once more the United States tried to pursue its agenda of getting cooperation for US consular inspections of departing vessels abroad. However, again it was rejected by a majority vote.[47] As we shall see, there were other issues of much greater significance discussed at the Rome conference, and the tensions that had been brewing in previous conferences bubbled over into both its scientific and political debates despite attempts to focus on practical matters. The *British Medical Journal* reported that as the conference prepared to commence, 'there will be a great temptation to some of the other Powers to introduce political questions into the discussions. If the conference is to be of any scientific value whatever, it will be needful that these should be rigidly excluded from the beginning.'[48] However, more than any previous conference, the sixth conference was politically motivated and arguably Britain's stance throughout was particularly so.

For the first time Britain had successfully argued for a separate Indian colonial (Raj) delegation, and after a brief postponement due to the fact that 'some opposition was made in certain quarters to the delegates of the Indian government being allowed to vote,'[49] the conference got under way on 20 May 1885. The delegates were carefully chosen. Richard Thorne Thorne represented Britain along with William Guyer-Hunter, who was Surgeon-General and who had led the official investigation into the cholera epidemic of 1883 that developed in Egypt only months after the British occupation. He had concluded that cholera was endemic to Egypt, that the epidemic had resulted from poisons in the soil, and that consequently it was not imported nor could it have been prevented with quarantines. His medical and political credentials were thus firmly established. The Government of India was similarly represented by known anti-quarantine physicians. Joseph Fayrer was President of the India Office Medical Board and a strong proponent of environmental theories of disease causation, while Timothy Richard Lewis had been a student of Pettenkofer and was 'special scientific assistant to the Indian government.'[50] As Harrison points out, 'Lewis and Fayrer were almost certainly chosen because of the congruence of their views with the political objectives of the Indian administration'; however, they were not 'untypical of medical opinion in India.'[51]

Within the first few days of the conference the medical delegates separated from the diplomatic representatives and formed what was known as the Technical Committee. Officially, the split was created to ensure the achievement of the conference's dual objectives: *technico-scientific* and *diplomatico-administrative*;[52] however, according to Thorne Thorne the origins of the Committee were more personal. When writing to his friend and superior, George Buchanan, he claimed that the Technical Committee was established both 'to prepare all the work and then to submit our conclusions to the Conference as a whole,' and because the elected president of the conference, a man named Cadorna who was President of the Italian Council of State, was thought to be a 'garrulous dotard, making a speech every time a delegate spoke and then proceeding to act the dictionary by giving lengthy expositions of the several words he had used'. Desiring an escape from the tedium, a 'conspiracy' was formed by several of the medical delegates against the man they considered an elderly bore and the Technical Committee emerged.[53]

With little pause the Committee lost sight of its 'technico-scientific' remit and became mired in political hostility. The timing of the Conference was critical. During the previous year the German Cholera Commission to India, led by Robert Koch, announced the 'discovery' of the causative agent of cholera, the *comma bacillus* or *vibrio cholerae*. However, reports and analyses of the Rome Conference in contemporary British medical journals exhibited little or no reference to the bacteriological aetiology of cholera and its impact on proceedings. Indeed, from the beginning the topic had been subverted at the conference, particularly in the Technical Committee where the British and Raj delegates blocked it from discussion. Fayrer, particularly, threatened to withdraw previous important votes he had made if 'questions of the aetiology of cholera and the theory of incubation were admitted to the discussion', particularly when Koch, who also served as Germany's medical delegate to the conference, began discussing the incubation period of cholera with regard to the bacillus.[54] The *Medical Times and Gazette*, a journal favoured among Britain's medical establishment and elite, proudly reported to its readers in June that

> the resolute determination of the British and Indian delegates, announced boldly from the first, to adhere to the question in its practical bearings, and abstain from all discussion on points opening up theoretical differences of opinion, was productive of good in many ways. It led to the avoidance of squabbling; it saved valuable time; it enabled the results of long practical experience to be put on record, and committed the Conference to no rash or ill considered action based upon *doubtful theoretical opinions which may not stand the test of time.*[55]

Seeking to avoid Koch's bacillus the British delegates, Thorne Thorne and Guyer-Hunter, tried to corral discussion of cholera to matters only of 'practical experience' such as clinical and epidemiological information and statistical documentation, which had underpinned previous critical British and Anglo-Indian studies on cholera.[56] Rather than representing 'objective' or 'apolitical' science, bacteriology was considered too controversial and provocative. Only by prohibiting it from the business of the Committee, Fayrer and his compatriot delegates argued, could sufficient conflict be avoided to enable profitable negotiations.

Part of what Koch's bacillus threatened to accuse, once more, was the role of Britain, in particular its role in India, in repeated European cholera epidemics. It was therefore essential to argue from the outset that cholera was not contagious, nor was it related in any way to shipping. Establishing this point, and the 'observable' science of epidemiology over laboratory based 'assumptions', Thorne Thorne and Fayrer challenged members of the conference to provide examples of British ships which had brought the disease directly from India to Europe or indeed any occasion where cholera had been introduced from Britain to Europe via shipping.[57] They demanded epidemiological evidence in support of notions of contagion which threatened to implicate Britain in the spread of cholera. As John Chapman, the physician and staunchly liberal proprietor and editor of the radical *Westminster Review*, wrote in his book on cholera published in the same year as the Rome conference:

> Dr Brouardel and Prout, representing France, insist, as many other members of the Congress do, that cholera always originates in India and that it is conveyed thence by means of ships to Europe, although no reply was given by any member of the Congress to Professor Lewis's inquiry whether any delegate knew of a single instance of cholera having been imported into Europe by an English ship; the non-contagionists, among whom were the English representatives, Professor Lewis and Sir William Guyer Hunter, affirm, if I am not mistaken, that cholera is capable of originating *de novo* in any locality where suitable conditions for its generation coexist, and that it is not brought from India to Europe, but that its foci of independent origin are probably as numerous in Europe and America as are the places in which it appears.[58]

Bacteriology and its 'contagious' implications were not open for debate. The British delegates were determined to exclude the laboratory in favour of clinical and epidemiological observation, citing numerous examples where cholera had failed to take root in efforts to refute the transmissibility of cholera via maritime trade links. Australia, they explained for example, had remained free from cholera despite its well-established trading links with India, omitting the crucial information that the Australian colonies enforced some of the most stringent of all quarantine systems.[59]

This was aetiology firmly rooted in Pettenkofer's theories and again it provided a comfortable compromise for Thorne Thorne and Fayrer to argue, for instance, that quarantine restrictions were worthless when compared with good 'local hygiene' which had proven successful in preventing cholera from 'taking root [in] the soil'.[60] Chapman summarised the opposing theories which, he believed, resulted in a conference that was 'heterogeneous and chaotic':

> one member of the Conference, representing Germany (Dr. Koch), affirms that a single comma-bacillus, gaining access to the alimentary canal of a man, is sufficient to kill him; another member, representing England, affirms that inasmuch as various microscopic organisms are found in cholera dejecta, the selection of the comma-shaped bacilli as the *materies morbi* of cholera appears to be entirely arbitrary, and that comma-shaped bacilli are ordinarily present in the mouths of healthy persons.[61]

These disagreements, however, were not merely about transmission but reflected competing practical and regulatory solutions to cholera, that in turn spoke to specific political interests, ideologies and rivalries, and situated very much at the centre of it all was the issue of how to control the potential flow of disease through the Suez Canal.

This was the first time that the issue of quarantine in the Canal had been raised at a conference. Surprisingly, the opening of the Canal was not mentioned at the 1874 conference in Vienna. Only five years after the Canal had opened in 1869, the epidemiological significance of this considerably faster route between India and Europe was not discussed, even though the conference had focused on India as the source of cholera, because it was assumed that existing inspection apparatuses in the Canal would be sufficient in the event of an epidemic.[62] Even so, the absence of the Canal in discussions at the Vienna conference is curious, while its constant role in the discussion at Rome was explosive. Considering the importance of the Canal in British, French and German imperial politics in the years leading up to 1885, it is not surprising that it became so absorbing.

In 1882, four years prior to the Rome conference, Egypt had effectively been made a quasi-protectorate of Britain after the British government had used military force to quell a nationalist uprising against increasing foreign influence. The armed response, and the command it subsequently allowed Britain to secure over the Canal, was not supported by the French who had previously shared control of Egypt's finances with Britain, leading to tensions between the two powers particularly over the Canal.

By 1885, nearly eighty per cent of the vessels which traversed the Canal each year were British. A large proportion of these sailed from Indian ports, principally Bombay, where cholera was undisputedly known to be endemic. What concerned most of the European nations represented at the Rome conference, however, was that unless the disease became 'epidemic', meaning that the number of cases rose beyond 'normal' levels, ships sailing from Indian ports were issued with clean Bills of Health. Thus, it was recommended that all ships which departed from India should be subject to prophylactic controls at Suez and it was proposed that an 'independent' medical officer, appointed by an international commission, would inspect all vessels intending to traverse the Canal. If a vessel was found to be 'infected' or 'suspected', all passengers and crew would be landed and it would be detained for five days under observation. The proposal was carried by a large majority but was vehemently opposed by the British and Raj delegates who argued that it called into question the objectivity and authority of the British medical officers who issued the Bills of Health in India. Thorne Thorne 'refused to allow that any locally appointed medical officer should supersede a British medical officer in deciding whether anyone on board an English ship was suspected of having some choleraic affection or not'.[63] Furthermore, he argued, any 'dirty and ill-kept' lazaretto maintained in Egypt was bound to be more hazardous to the spread of disease than the free pratique of a well-sanitised British vessel.[64] The latter, it was implied, were part of the larger complex of the 'English' sanitary zone, emblematically secure and approved for unhindered passage. It was nonsensical, Thorne Thorne and his fellow compatriot and imperial delegates insisted, to impose quarantines or other restrictions in the Suez Canal, or elsewhere on the route from India. Instead, they argued, what was required were sanitary improvements and measures similar to those which had been introduced 'at home', expanding the 'sanitary zone' and reinforcing British influence in the newly secured territory around the Canal.

Although often using the language of medical or sanitary science, cholera prevention became almost a secondary issue to the more immediate political issues surrounding the Canal. The simultaneous proceeding of the Suez Canal International Commission in Paris had particular bearing on the way the Canal was discussed in relation to cholera. It had come together primarily in response to French and Russian concerns about the use of the Canal after the British occupation of Egypt and the increasing international desire to assure its 'neutrality'. However, both the Paris Commission and the Rome Conference became venues in which the tensions between France and Britain over Egypt could be played out. As an editorial in *The Times* observed:

> It is impossible not to discern a political connexion, more or less direct and certainly not without grave significance, between the proposals adopted by the Committee of the Sanitary Conference, mainly at the insistence of the French delegates, and the provisions of the draft treaty at present under consideration of the Suez Canal Commission now sitting in Paris. In both cases may be traced the working of that unfriendly and unaccommodating spirit towards this country which has long pervaded the Egyptian policy of France, and now seems to have *infected* the policy of other European Powers.[65]

France, particularly, was wary of supporting Britain's interests in the Canal, angered by Britain's unilateral termination of British and French dual control of Egypt, and along with many other nations, was particularly apprehensive about the Canal being reduced to an appendage of the British Empire.[66] The Paris convention was thus convened with the purpose of reaffirming the international character of the Canal and asserting its neutral status with the establishment of an international Canal Commission. Britain strongly opposed this, wanting instead to limit the restraints of international control which they anticipated would hinder free movement through the Canal. However, at the Paris Commission as at the Sanitary Conference, Britain was alone in its plans for the Canal, and a convention, 'largely directed against Britain', was drawn up in early summer 1885, imposing international laws upon passage through the Canal.[67] Much of the deliberations at the Paris meeting were led by the French and the animosity felt between France and Britain in Paris was mirrored in the proceedings at Rome.

Thorne Thorne, who kept regular correspondence with Buchanan, Chief Medical Officer of the Local Government Board, wrote often about the hostility he felt from the French representatives, and the highly politicised nature of the discussions of the Technical Committee. He wrote:

> It was quite intelligible ... that Austria, Italy and other countries in close proximity to Egyptian ports should, under the apprehension of cholera and in view of the exaggerated opinions held by their population on the subject, be desirous of the enforcement in Egypt of extreme measures

or precaution for the relief and security of their outposts. But I did not understand how it should happen that the French Representatives should be the prime movers in advocating a system of observance and quarantine which if rigidly carried out would probably have the effect of driving British commerce with the East to take the route round the Cape of Good Hope to the detriment of the Suez Canal in which France had such an interest.[68]

British medical journals and newspapers reporting on the Rome conference reported a general motivation among those countries represented at the conference, particularly France, who supported quarantine in the Canal, as attempting to arrogate political advantage by trying to 'fetter ... in some degree our great Indian commerce'.[69] It was also widely reported, with a twinge of wounded bewilderment, that numerous European powers believed that Britain's objection to quarantine in the Suez Canal was motivated purely by commercial concerns.[70] This was not merely the result of British neurosis; France and Germany, particularly, were convinced of the British commercial motivations behind the objections to quarantine, as this translated extract from *Marseille Medical* demonstrates:

> The English, who are protected by their climate from the influence of cholera – the English aristocracy of which forms a class apart, and which knows well that by means of hygiene and comfort (when they are to be had) it is possible to ensure safety from cholera, ... would consent *without compunction* [*sans douleur*] that the whole universe should enjoy the benefits of endemic cholera, provided that every obstacle to the transport of their products be removed ...[71]

Clearly then, many of the debates and resolutions of the Rome conference were more related to political demands and reactions concerning relations between Britain, Europe and the Canal, than they were with the pursuit of internationally agreed methods of cholera prevention. Regardless of whether the central focus was concerned with political control of the thoroughfare, as at Paris or as at Rome, the epidemiological and medical effects of this speedier route between Europe and South and East Asia, the issues and responses were the same. Britain argued for the maintenance of (its own) free movement either through limiting international control or through preserving the free pratique of British ships sailing from all ports; while France, for example and for a variety of reasons, not least being to obstruct British interests, wished to see these restrictions imposed on Canal traffic.

Commercial pressures on Britain to ensure the limitation of costly delays in the Canal were immense. While both the Rome and Paris conferences were taking place, complaints were voiced by companies such as the influential Peninsular and Oriental Steam Navigation Company about quarantine at Suez, and by 'the principal Eastern steamship lines' who held a meeting in London:

> concerning measures for the protection of their interests, and it was resolved by them to amend their bills of lading in order that on the imposition of quarantine steamers homeward bound from an infected port should be at liberty to proceed by way of the Cape, and so avoid delay at Suez. It is found by experience that in the case of large vessels of modern construction the loss of time by the Cape is almost compensated for by the saving of the canal dues, and that a few days' detention at Suez would remove all advantages now existing in favour of that route.[72]

However, while interest in the Rome conference and discussions surrounding its possible implications were the topic of numerous shipping company meetings and journal and newspaper articles and editorials, there was no mention of the highly contentious proceedings of the International Sanitary Conference at Rome in the Port of London Sanitary Committee papers or minutes in 1885. Nor did the Committee discuss Koch's work. That Koch's 'discovery' of the cholera bacillus was not mentioned is perhaps not so surprising. If the British and Raj medical delegates at the conference refused to speak of it even in Koch's presence and with other European and American delegates eager to discuss its implications, it is not so difficult to understand why the domestic sanitary authorities in Britain did not feel it necessary to introduce into their business. However, that an international conference, singularly concerned with cholera prophylaxis at major ports and having particular relevance to the arrival of infected ships from Britain's colonies, was not mentioned in the papers of Britain's principal – and central – Port Sanitary Committee is quite surprising. Since the Committee was, under ordinary circumstances, in regular correspondence with Richard Thorne Thorne, it might be expected that some news of Rome would be found in the papers; but, no special correspondence regarding the conference was received from him, or anyone else – although Thorne Thorne had written to Buchanan throughout his time in Rome.[73]

Some of the proposals made by the British and colonial Indian delegates at the conference had direct and important ramifications for

British ports. It was, for example, proposed that rather than imposing quarantine on British ships as they traversed the Suez Canal, these vessels could sail through without having contact with the shore; that they 'should always be allowed to pass through the Suez Canal as through an arm of the sea'.[74] If the ships sailed directly to Britain from India without having contact with the shore, quarantine, they argued, would not be necessary. As Thorne Thorne explained:

> We maintained that no British vessel passing from India to England had ever yet conveyed cholera to Europe, and hence that we could not, merely because other countries did not wish vessels from the East to enter their ports without first undergoing a period of detention, admit the right of anyone to say that British vessels coming to our ports and touching nowhere else should be otherwise than unhindered in their course.[75]

However, this would in effect have meant that ships from 'infected ports' – as cholera was endemic in ports such as Bombay and Calcutta – would arrive in London having had no quarantine or even disinfection since it had embarked. While the incubation period was believed to have been less than the time taken for the journey from India, no definitive interval had been agreed upon. Even so, this issue – the arrival of vessels directly from India – was similarly absent from Committee discussions, as were discussions about the incubation period of cholera. Similarly, the possibility that the conference could have resulted in an international convention requiring minimum and maximum periods of quarantine at all ports into which 'infected' or 'suspected' ships sailed – ships from India, for instance – had direct relevance for the workings of the Sanitary Committee, yet also remained unmentioned.

Even though Britain did not experience a cholera epidemic between 1872 and 1892, cholera featured as an important issue in British ports in the mid-1880s. The committee papers and minutes of the Port Sanitary Committee clearly demonstrate, in contrast to the attitudes expressed by British delegates at the Rome conference, an anxiety about the presence of cholera in Italy, Spain and France, and the almost certain 'recrudescence of cholera on the Continent' anticipated in the spring/summer of 1885.[76] These concerns were compounded by the arrival of various ships from India, during 1884 and 1885, which reached England having endured a number of cases of cholera on board during their voyage. Yet, it was because the Committee and Medical Officers knew that vessels which came from India had invariably undergone quarantine and disinfection before reaching England that they were not too anxious when they arrived. Reporting on one such 'infected' vessel, the preventive systems of other States, including quarantine, that punctuated the journey from Asia, appeared to mitigate any unease:

> On the 29th May, owing to an intimation from the Customs, I visited the *S.S. Nivia* from Calcutta, one of the crew on board having died from cholera during the voyage – The death occurred on 20th April, the corpse was at once buried at sea and the bedding, clothing and everything used by the deceased during his illness destroyed – on arriving at Ceylon the passengers were landed and the ship was thoroughly fumigated and disinfected – Again on reaching Port Said the passengers were put on shore, the ship was placed in Quarantine for seven days, fumigated and disinfected twice over – There was no other case of infectious disease on board during the voyage – *Under these circumstances* no further sanitary action was deemed necessary – the vessel was released and saved her tide up the River.[77]

Another ship, *The Queen of Scots*, arrived into Gravesend from Calcutta in September 1885 with the clothes of a man who had died of cholera on board and, conversely, showed the anxiety attendant with a lack of remote quarantine. As the disease had been present in the 'homeward' passage, it was deemed infectious and 'ought therefore to have been detained at Gravesend', but, as the disease – or the clothes – had not been reported, the master of the vessel was fined £20 and the Committee set about establishing measures which would ensure such an occurrence was not repeated.

Thus, the absence, in Port Sanitary Committee correspondence, of any discussion about proposals put to the 1885 conference regarding the passage of vessels direct from India to Britain is peculiar. The Port of London Sanitary Authority only appeared to be at ease with the *S.S. Nivia* because it was clear that she had already undergone extensive disinfection and a period of quarantine on the homeward journey, while *The Queen of Scots* caused such a stir because it had not. The implication, therefore and in agreement with Baldwin's theory of 'geoepidemiology',[78] is that part of the ease which the English System displayed in dealing with such cases was due to the knowledge that, in most cases, vessels from Asian ports had already undergone one, if not several, period(s) of isolation and disinfection before they reached Britain. The absence in the Port Sanitary Committee papers and minutes of any reference to the conference, or the proposal made by British delegates to have vessels sail directly from India without docking, suggests either that they were unaware of the deliberations of the conference, despite considerable press coverage, or that the day-to-day running of the ports demanded all of their attention. Perhaps one may also speculate that the Port authorities did not anticipate any agreement on the matter. The conference was widely believed to be stacked in favour of quarantine and against British interests, and it was well known that Britain would not endorse any international agreement calling for minimum periods of medical detention. In terms of the practical operation of disease control at domestic ports, the likelihood of change was minimal. And these assumptions turned out to be well founded, as the Rome conference was again unable to produce a ratified agreement and quarantine continued to operate on a nation-to-nation basis.

'A dangerous and unverifiable statement...'

Britain's reluctance to enter into any discussion regarding a specific causative agent for cholera at the 1885 conference followed the pattern of previous conferences where it consistently stood apart from other European States in its total allegiance to the non-contagious nature of cholera and other imported diseases. While this did not necessarily reflect general approaches to aetiological theory in Britain or the way that bacteriology or Koch's 'discovery' was received among British physicians as a whole, it remained at the heart of port health. In this arena, environmental factors, as suggested by Pettenkofer who was still regarded in the late 1880s as 'the greatest living authority on the aetiology of cholera',[79] continued to play a more prominent role in aetiological thinking. Koch's theory was at odds with this, asserting that the *comma bacillus* was the singular cause of cholera and that environment played no 'miasmatic' role in the spread of the disease.

Koch's *vibrio cholerae* was discovered while 'Germany's leading bacteriologist' was working for the German Cholera Commission in Calcutta in 1884.[80] Despite the acclaim Koch received in Berlin after it was announced that he had discovered the cause of the disease, his assertion that the *comma bacillus* was the source of cholera could not be proven using his own tightly defined methodology. Since the 1870s, a sequence of rules dictating the necessary criteria for determining whether a particular micro-organism was the cause of a disease had been clearly laid out by Koch's teacher at the University of Göttingen, Jakob Helne, and refined by Koch himself. These were known as 'Koch's Postulates' and they asserted that: first, an organism must be shown to be present in all who suffer from the disease and absent from those who do not; it then needs to be isolated and reproduced in the laboratory in a pure culture; from this, a healthy animal must be infected, reproducing the disease from which organisms identical to the original can be reisolated.

However, the main weakness in Koch's argument was that although the bacillus found in the intestines of cholera victims was isolated and a pure culture produced, he was unable to reproduce the disease in animals. So, although he successfully demonstrated the existence of the bacillus and its association with cholera, he did not fulfil his own criteria for categorically proving that the organism was the *cause* of the disease. Instead, he left open the possibility that the *comma bacillus* could simply have been a *consequence* of cholera.[81] It was this shortcoming which encouraged much of the scientific opposition to Koch's findings in Britain. Edward Klein, the notable London-based bacteriologist who along with Heneage Gibbs conducted the English Cholera Commission in India to examine Koch's findings, noted that 'with few exceptions most Continental pathologists consider the comma bacilli of Koch as being the cause of cholera'. However, he claimed, 'most' British physicians and scientists working on the disease 'differ from the proposition that Koch's comma bacilli have been satisfactorily proved to be the cause of cholera', and that the 'prevailing opinion [was] that the comma bacilli of Koch [were only] an important diagnostic guide'.[82]

While a number of prominent British physicians such as Joseph Lister and Edgar Crookshank responded enthusiastically to news of Koch's bacillus, many British physicians, particularly Medical Officers of Health and those at the Local Government Board, continued to argue that epidemiological and clinical experience demonstrated the close association between environment and disease and that the methods of prophylaxis developed and employed according to these theories were successful in preventing the spread of disease.[83] Demonstrating this point, Sir William Gull, physician extraordinary to the Queen, observed that 'we may in fact be able to defend ourselves against the invasion of cholera before science has discovered the essential cause of the disease. This happened very largely in the case of ague [malaria], where, by drainage and other matters, the occurrence of miasmata has been prevented'.[84] Gull's argument was well received when he presented it to twelve other physicians at the India Office. They had all been invited to form a committee there to discuss the published results of Klein and Gibbs's investigations in India titled 'An Inquiry into the Etiology of Asiatic Cholera'. In response to this document, they were asked to discuss the scientific value and validity of Koch's 'discovery'. Their conclusions were published in a report called, unambiguously, 'The Official Refutation of Dr. Robert Koch's Theory of Cholera and Commas', in which Koch's 'discovery' was rejected on several grounds.[85] These included: firstly, that the bacillus could not be used to reproduce cholera in lower animals; secondly, that comma shaped bacilli were said to be ordinarily present in the alimentary tract of healthy people; and because water tanks which had been contaminated with the faeces of cholera victims, and contained the *comma bacillus*, had failed to produce cholera in the villagers who consumed the water.[86]

Yet, a bacteriological classification and aetiology for cholera was resisted not only because of its apparent scientific shortcomings; it also had important implications for the policy and practice of public health and port prophylaxis. The connection was clear. In the closing statement of 'The Official Refutation' the committee declared that it could not end without clearly stating that quarantines were 'positively injurious' and created 'unavoidable hardships' as well as unnecessary alarm, while 'sanitary measures alone, are the only trustworthy means to prevent outbreaks of the disease'.[87] The unmistakable implication was that Koch's bacillus threatened to undermine the local and environmental theories that created and supported the sanitary system. It was, within this context, potentially quite a 'dangerous' idea:

> The doctrine of contagion ... is still maintained by many influential authorities on the Continent and here; the former loudly insisting on quarantine and charging us with conniving at the introduction of cholera to Europe, rather than interfere with our own mercantile interests ... That a bacillus in association with cholera has been detected there need be no question ... but that the cause of cholera has been discovered any more than it was before ... I believe to be a dangerous and unverifiable statement, inasmuch as it will tend to emphasise the views of contagion and the importance of quarantine already so much insisted upon.[88]

Within the context of port health, it was the theoretical implications of a specific causative agent, rather than the microbe necessarily, which were considered highly problematic. Whether before or after the culpable microbe had been identified, the theoretical basis of bacteriology was associated with 'old-school' contagionism, which allowed for the transmission of disease irrespective of environment. Regardless of whether Koch's 'discovery' was considered legitimate or not – when measured against Koch's postulates – the *comma bacillus* was essentially less problematic than an acceptance of the theoretical basis of his findings. An acceptance of the 'contagionism' that underlay bacteriology, 'proven' or 'unproven', meant an acceptance of the principles of quarantine. This was clearly demonstrated in the reaction of the British and Indian colonial delegates at the 1885 Rome conference. It was also evident within the vast number of publications, of greater and lesser medical content, which emerged in relation to issues of port health in the period after 1883.

Rather than fading, this rejection of the *vibrio cholerae* endured at the highest levels of the British and imperial medical hierarchy for several years. The scribbled notes of a meeting held at the Royal College of Physicians in London in May 1889 illustrate with particular clarity the continued hostility to Koch's *comma bacillus* in the years following the 'discovery'. The Colonial Office, with an attached dispatch from the Governor of Barbados, had approached the Royal College with an inquiry as to the appropriate 'periods of detention for purposes of Quarantine in Yellow Fever, Cholera and Small-pox'. True to form, the assembled Committee of four influential physicians, including Fayrer as well as Thomas Graham Balfour who had been the Surgeon-General of the British Army and was, by 1889, President of the Royal Statistical Society, delivered its conclusions in a one-page report, stating:

> That the incubation period of Yellow Fever and Cholera is uncertain, and the Committee is of opinion that it is unwise to impose Quarantine restrictions in the case of these diseases.
>
> The Committee is further strongly opposed to such restrictions generally, which it considers harmful and vexatious.[89]

Most illuminating, however, are the barely legible and anonymous short-hand notes written during the meeting and scratched onto the back of a printed letter of invitation. They reveal the strong aversion to a bacterial cause of cholera developed among many high-level physicians in Britain in the years immediately following the 'discovery' of the *comma bacillus*. As might be expected from a committee attended by Fayrer, quarantine was harshly opposed. Indeed the notes begin with Fayrer calling for a 'general protest against Quarantine'. The committee discussed how it would be 'absurd to Quar[antine] a ship wh[ich] comes f[rom] an infected place and one wh[ich] has chol[era] on board', and that, 'all precautions except sanitary ones and medical inspection are useless, these precautions should be such as are adopted in this country & not suffering the laws of Quarantine'. These comments are perhaps predictable, yet the few comments relating to the incubation period and cause of cholera and yellow fever are what particularly stand out in the notes. According to these eminent fellows of the Royal College, 'the incub[ation] period of Yell[ow] fev[er] & chol[era] is undefined/uncertain & the cause'. Considering that the meeting took place in 1889, six years after the announcement of Koch's cholera bacillus, and the subsequent acceptance of the theory on the Continent, the statement was particularly pointed. Rather, all the members of the committee rejected bacterial contagion and concurred that the diseases were 'affected by climate – just as is affected in sewerage'. The notes concluded with Fayrer:

Sir J. Fayrer.
They wanted to do away with Quar[antine] in Roman conference –
Thorne & I & Hunter opposed it – & to good effect.
    Others wanted to return to the ...[?]... System. Whole of Europe deranged by fear of bacillus – Koch did all that.[90]

Clearly the matter was not easily resolved. After the moderate headway made by Britain in reducing European reliance on quarantine during the 1874 conference, the announcement of a specific contagious agent in 1883 appeared to have had a regressive effect. It became much more difficult for British physicians to argue, in an international forum, that the maintenance of a sanitary urban environment could provide sufficient protection from epidemic cholera after a germ had been identified which could, theoretically, produce the disease regardless of local conditions.

Variations on a localist aetiology for cholera, however, were not only maintained because they suited Britain's commercial and political interests, but they were also well supported by substantial epidemiological investigations undertaken by prominent physicians in both Britain and India.[91] Furthermore, experience had demonstrated overwhelmingly after the 1866 epidemic that public health reforms, including the English System from 1872, sufficed in precluding any great extension of the disease from individual cases which arrived into the ports. At the same time, it appeared that the 'unsanitary' ports and lazarettos of the subcontinent, Lavant and Mediterranean were culpable, rather than any infective agent, for their numerous and devastating epidemics of cholera. The argument continued to be made that observation, rather than laboratory science, had already provided the answer. Non-contagionism, exemplified by the rejection of the *vibrio cholerae*, was thus not merely maintained because it endorsed the commercial requirements of free trade and movement, but also because it was supported by half a century of epidemiological investigations, clinical research and experience. And in addition to all of these compelling reasons to continue, at least in relation to port health, non-contagionist thinking about cholera, the careers and personal reputations of a number of prominent individuals had also been hinged on the promotion of localist theories. In sum, too much was at stake.

Conclusion

Yet, even with these strong political and medical objections to and arguments against quarantine, it continued to endure as a legal, and to an extent practical, barrier at British ports until 1896. How can this be explained when none of the conferences until the 1890s resulted in a ratified agreement? Britain was free to perform any means of disease prevention it chose within its own ports, and could without legal recourse have easily removed all vestiges of the much despised quarantine earlier in the century. However, the interconnectedness of international ports, travel and commerce prohibited such unilateral action. While other States continued to rely on quarantine, Britain could not be seen to abandon it entirely if British ships were to continue to participate fully and effectively in international trade. According to most European States, a port such as London, for example, if it did not have a legal requirement to quarantine ships suspected of carrying 'exotic' disease, would have been considered an 'infected' port. This would have meant that all ships from London would consequently be deemed suspicious and probably quarantined when they sailed into foreign ports. Driven by imperial rivalry, many States would have been delighted at the opportunity to enforce such a hindrance to Britain's maritime dominance. And so, while it might have been acknowledged that in practice Britain protected her ports almost entirely with sanitary measures, officially quarantine remained as a legal obligation and was still required of ships infected with any of the 'exotic' diseases, plague, yellow fever or cholera, which arrived into British ports.

In order, therefore, to reconcile international pressures with national interests, the system of dual authority which accommodated both a sanitary and quarantine response to imported disease was established at the ports in 1872. With the creation of the Port Sanitary Authorities, the arrival of cholera was managed essentially with sanitary rather than quarantine measures, addressing the source of the disease principally within the urban environment and the 'English' sanitary zone, but responding at the same time to international pressures that compelled Britain to maintain even just a nominal quarantine.

It is here then that we see the consequence of foreign pressures on British domestic policy, and the significance of the ports as an interface between foreign and domestic policy and practice is clearly illustrated. British physicians in charge of controlling the import of infectious disease into domestic, and some imperial, ports could not overlook the opinions and demands of foreign – principally European – States in the design or implementation of prophylaxis, regardless of their medical or political convictions. The fact that the 1825 Quarantine Act remained law, despite the apparent success of the Port Sanitary Authorities after 1872 and the obvious difficulties which lay in dual authority, was largely a consequence of the force of international compulsion, clearly demonstrated at the International Sanitary Conferences. The exigency of accommodating, within British domestic policy, the overwhelming desire of European powers to quarantine was essential if Britain, despite its naval and imperial supremacy at the end of the nineteenth century, was to participate more or less unhindered in international trade. Thus, paradoxically, in order for Britain to maintain freedom of movement of British ships and trade around the world, it had to maintain, domestically, the one system which embodied exactly the opposite of this.

Table 2.1 Representative states at the International Sanitary Conferences, 1851–1907[92]

First Conference – Paris, 23 July 1851–19 January 1852
Austria, the Two Sicilies, Spain, the Papal States, France, Great Britain, Greece, Portugal, Russia, Sardinia, Tuscany and Turkey

Second Conference – Paris, 9 April 1859–30 August 1859
Austria, France, Great Britain, Greece, the Papal States, Portugal, Russia, Sardinia, Spain, Tuscany and Turkey. Representatives of the Ionian Islands were sent as observers.

Third Conference – Constantinople, 13 February 1866–26 September 1866
Austria, Belgium, Denmark, France, Spain, the Papal States, Great Britain, Greece, Italy, Netherlands, Persia, Portugal, Prussia, Russia, Sweden and Norway (then political unified) and Turkey. The United States was invited but did not attend. Egypt, the under Turkish Sovereignty, observed.

Fourth Conference – Vienna, 1 July 1874–1 August 1874
Austria-Hungary, Belgium, Denmark, Egypt, France, Germany, Great Britain, Greece, Italy, Luxembourg, Netherlands, Norway, Persia, Portugal, Roumania, Russia, Serbia, Spain, Sweden, Switzerland and Turkey. The United States was invited but did not attend.

Fifth Conference – Washington, 5 January 1881–1 March 1881
Argentina, Austria-Hungary, Belgium, Bolivia, Brazil, Chile, China, Colombia, Denmark, France, Germany, great Britain, Hawaii, Haiti, Italy, Japan, Liberia, Mexico, Netherlands, Portugal, Russia, Spain, Sweden and Norway, Turkey, the United States and Venezuela. Canada and Cuba with Porto Rico sent medical delegates only.

Sixth Conference – Rome, 20 May 1885–13 June 1885
Argentina, Austria-Hungary, Belgium, Brazil, Chile, China, Denmark, France, Germany, Great Britain, Greece, Guatemala, India, Italy, Japan, Mexico, Netherlands, Peru, Portugal, Roumania, Russia, Serbia, Spain, Sweden and Norway, Switzerland, Turkey, the United States and Uruguay. Egypt is given as attending although did not send a delegate.

Seventh Conference – Venice, 5–31 January 1892
Austria-Hungary, Belgium, Denmark, France, Germany, Great Britain, Greece, Italy, Netherlands, Portugal, Russia, Spain, Sweden and Norway and Turkey (including Egypt). Representatives of the Quarantine Board at Alexandria were also sent.

Eighth Conference – Dresden, 11 March 1893–15 April 1893
Austria-Hungary, Belgium, Denmark, France, Germany, Great Britain, Greece, Italy, Luxembourg, Montenegro, Netherlands, Portugal, Roumania, Russia, Spain, Serbia, Sweden and Norway, Switzerland and Turkey.

Table 2.1 (Continued)

Ninth Conference – Paris, 7 February 1894–3 April 1894
Austria-Hungary, Belgium, Denmark, France, Germany, Great Britain,
Greece, Italy, Netherlands, Persia, Portugal, Russia, Spain, Serbia, Turkey and
the United States.

Tenth Conference – Venice, 16 February 1897–19 March 1897
Austria-Hungary, Belgium, Denmark, France, Germany, Great Britain,
Greece, Italy, Luxembourg, Montenegro, Netherlands, Portugal, Roumania,
Russia, Spain, Serbia, Sweden and Norway, Switzerland and Turkey. Bulgaria
and Egypt were also present although not 'officially' independent.

Eleventh Conference – Paris, 10 October 1903–3 December 1903
Argentina, Austria-Hungary, Belgium, Brazil, Denmark, France, Germany,
Great Britain, Greece, Italy, Luxembourg, Montenegro, Netherlands, Persia,
Portugal, Roumania, Russia, Serbia, Spain, Sweden and Norway, Switzerland,
Turkey and the United States.

L'Office International d'Hygiene publique – 'The Paris Office' – 1907
Establishment of first permanent, worldwide body dealing with
international health – primarily quarantine.

Notes

1 Valeska Huber, 'The Unifaction of the Globe by Disease? The International
 Sanitary Conferences on Cholera, 1851–1894,' *The Historical Journal*, 49,
 2 (2006), 453–76, pp. 455–6.
2 Baldwin, *Contagion and the State*, p. 149.
3 Ackerknecht, 'Anticontagionism,' 562–93.
4 Christopher Hamlin, 'Commentary: Ackerknecht and "Anticontagionism":
 A Tale of Two Dichotomies,' *International Journal of Epidemiology*, 38
 (2009), 22–7, p. 22; and Charles Rosenberg, 'Commentary: Epidemiology
 in Context,' *International Journal of Epidemiology*, 38 (2009), 28–30,
 p. 30.
5 Ackerknecht, 'Anticontagionism,' p. 589 (original italics).
6 *Ibid.*, p. 567 (original italics).
7 *Ibid.*
8 For example: Pelling, *Cholera, Fever and English Medicine*; and Cooter,
 'Anticontagionism and History's Medical Record,' pp. 87–108.
9 Baldwin, *Contagion and the State*, p. 563.
10 Worboys, *Spreading Germs*, pp. 35–6.
11 *Ibid.*, p. 148.
12 George Buchanan, 'Precautions against Cholera', *Fourteenth Annual
 Report of the LGB, 1884–5 – Supplement Containing the Report of the*

Medical Officer (London: Eyre and Spottiswoode, 1885), Appendix A, p. 24 [C. 4516] (original emphasis).

13 Ackerknecht, 'Anticontagionism', pp. 569.

14 Worboys, *Spreading Germs,* pp. 109–10.

15 *Ibid.,* p. 131.

16 Jeremy Isaacs, 'D.D. Cunningham and the Aetiology of Cholera in British India, 1869–1897', *Medical History,* 42 (1998), 279–305, pp. 291–4; Harrison, *Public Health,* pp. 111–16; Sheldon Watts, 'Cholera Politics in Britain in 1879: John Netten Radcliffe's Confidential Memo on "Quarantine in the Red Sea",' *The Journal of the Historical Society,* 7, 3 (2007), 291–411.

17 See Table 2.1 for full list of representatives at this and subsequent conferences to 1907.

18 Mark Harrison, 'Disease, Diplomacy and International Commerce: The Origins of International Sanitary Regulation in the Nineteenth Century,' *Journal of Global History,* 1, 2 (2006), 197–217, p. 213.

19 World Health Organisation (WHO), *The First Ten Years of the World Health Organisation* (Geneva: World Health Organisation, 1958), p. 6.

20 *Ibid.,* pp. 6–7.

21 The medical and diplomatic representatives of each country had a separate vote. Very often the two representatives voted differently, essentially cancelling out the vote of that nation. This problem was rectified in later conferences by allowing only one vote per country.

22 Neville M. Goodman, *International Health Organisations and Their Work* (Edinburgh: Churchill Livingstone, 1971), p. 44.

23 WHO, *The First Ten Years,* p. 10; see also Worboys, *Spreading Germs,* p. 38.

24 N. Howard–Jones, 'The Scientific Background of the International Sanitary Conferences, 1851–1938. 1' *WHO Chronicle,* 28 (1974), 159–71, p. 162.

25 *General Board of Health–Report on the Epidemic Cholera of 1848–49.* House of Commons Parliamentary Papers (1850), 21, 1273–75.

26 Stephen Halliday, 'Commentary: Dr John Sutherland, Vibrio Cholerae and 'Predisposing Causes,"' *International Journal of Epidemiology,* 31, 5 (2002), 912–14; see also, Watts, 'Cholera Politics.'

27 Howard-Jones, 'The Scientific Background… 1', p. 164.

28 J. Lane Notter, 'International Sanitary Conferences of the Victorian Era', *Transactions of the Epidemiological Society of London,* XVII (1897–98), 1–14, p. 2.

29 Amir Arsalan Afkami, 'Defending the Guarded Domain: Epidemics and the Emergence of an International Sanitary Policy in Iran,' *Comparative Studies of South Asia, Africa and the Middle East,* 19, 1 (1999), 122–34, p. 124.

30 Howard-Jones, 'The Scientific Background... 2', *WHO Chronicle,* 28 (1974), 229–47, p. 236.

31 Harrison, *Public Health,* p. 118.

32 E. Goodeve, 'On the International Sanitary Conference, and the Preservation of Europe from Cholera', *Transactions of the Epidemiological Society of London,* III (1866–67), 15–31.

33 *Report to the International Sanitary Conference of a Commission from That Body, to Which Were Referred the Questions Relative to the Origin, Endemicity, Transmissibility and Propagation of Asiatic Cholera* (Translated by Samuel L. Abbott) (London: Alfred Mudge & Son, 1867), p. 86.

34 Isaacs, 'D.D. Cunningham,' p. 282.

35 Baldwin, *Contagion and the State,* p. 143.

36 Pelling, *Cholera, Fever and English Medicine,* pp. 247–8; Worboys, *Spreading Germs,* p. 115.

37 Mark Harrison, 'A Question of Locality: The Identity of Cholera in British India, 1860–1890', in D. Arnold (ed.), *Warm Climate and Western Medicine: The Emergence of Tropical Medicine, 1500–1900* (Amsterdam: Rodopi, 1996), 133–59, p. 144.

38 Quoted in Howard-Jones, 'The Scientific Background... 2', pp. 243–4.

39 Sir Richard Thorne Thorne (1841–99) became a supernumerary inspector in the medical department of the Privy Council in 1868, and in this capacity he conducted several investigations in connection with outbreaks of typhoid fever with such marked ability that in February 1871 he was appointed a permanent inspector. He rose gradually from this position until in 1892 he succeeded to the post of principal medical officer to the Local Government Board on the retirement of Sir George Buchanan.

Thorne's knowledge of French and German, 'no less than his polished manners and courtly address', soon made him especially acceptable to his political chiefs, and he was repeatedly selected to represent his country in matters of international hygiene. Thus he was the British delegate at the International Sanitary Conferences held at Rome in 1885, at Venice in 1892, at Dresden in 1893, at Paris in 1894, at Venice in 1897; and was Her Majesty's plenipotentiary to sign the conventions of Dresden in 1893, Paris in 1894, and Venice in 1897, the last convention being very largely drawn up under his guidance.

Dictionary of National Biography, Suppl. Vol. 3 (1901), p. 382; 'Obituary', *Transactions of the Epidemiological Society of London,* XIX (1899–1900), p. 210.

40 R. Thorne Thorne, 'On the Result of the International Sanitary Conference of Rome, 1885', *Transactions of the Epidemiological Society of London,* V (1885–86), pp. 135–49, p. 144.

41 *National Board of Health Bulletin,* vol. 2, no. 7, 14 August 1880 (Washington), p. 485.

42 Howard-Jones, 'The Scientific Background... 3', 369–84, p. 370.

43 *National Board of Health Bulletin*, vol. 1, no. 1, 28 June 1979 (Washington), p. 3.

44 Howard-Jones, 'The Scientific Background... 3', 369–84, p. 370.

45 *Proceedings of the International Sanitary Conference Provided for by Joint Resolution of the Senate and House of Representatives in the Early Part of 1881* (Washington: Government Printing Office, 1881), p. 16.

46 Goodman, *International Health Organisations*, p. 62; see also chapter 4.

47 *Medical Times and Gazette* (London), 30 May 1885, p. 734.

48 *BMJ*, 4 April 1885, vol. 1, p. 708.

49 *BMJ*, 16 May 1885, vol. 1, p. 1013.

50 Harrison, *Public Health*, p. 56; see also Isaacs, 'D.D. Cunningham'; and Mariko Ogawa, "Uneasy Bedfellows: Science and Politics in the Refutation of Koch's Bacterial Theory of Cholera", *Bulletin of the History of Medicine*, 74 (2000), 671–707, p. 692.

51 Harrison, *Public Health*, p. 127.

52 Howard-Jones, 'The Scientific Background... 3', p. 382.

53 Letter dated, 25 May 1885, NA, MH113/22.

54 Howard-Jones, 'The Scientific Background... 3', p. 382.

55 *Medical Times and Gazette*, 20 June 1885, p. 820 (my italics).

56 Sheldon Watts, 'Cholera and the Maritime Environment of Great Britain, India and the Suez Canal: 1866–1883,' *International Journal of Environmental Studies*, 63, 1 (2006) 19–38; and Watts, 'Cholera Politics.'

57 Joseph Fayrer, *Recollections of My Life* (London: William Blackwood and Sons, 1900), p. 452.

58 John Chapman, *Cholera Curable: A Demonstration of the Causes, Non-Contagiousness, and Successful Treatment of the Disease* (London: Churchill, 1885), pp. 85–6.

59 *The Lancet*, 6 June 1885, vol. 1, p. 1053; see also, Krista Maglen, 'A World Apart: Geography, Australian Quarantine, and the Mother Country', *Journal of the History of Medicine and Allied Sciences*, 60, 2 (2005), 196–217.

60 *BMJ*, 13 June 1885, vol. 1, p. 1222.

61 Chapman, *Cholera Curable*, p. 85.

62 Harrison, *Public Health*, p. 119.

63 *BMJ*, 16 May 1885, vol. 1, p. 1013.

64 Howard-Jones, 'The Scientific Background... 3', p. 383.

65 *The Times*, 2 June 1885, p. 9d.

66 D.A. Farnie, *East and West of Suez – The Suez Canal in History, 1854–1956* (Oxford: Clarendon Press, 1969), p. 329.

67 *Ibid.*, p. 330.

68 Letter dated, 3 June 1885, NA, MH113/22.

69 *Medical Times and Gazette*, 13 June 1885, p. 798.

70 See for example: *Medical Times and Gazette,* 6 June 1885, p. 747; *BMJ,* June 13, 1885, p. 1222; *The Times,* 2 June 1885, p. 9d.

71 *Marseille Medical,* 30 October 1884, in Chapman, *Cholera Curable,* p. 87.

72 *The Times,* 12 June 1885, p. 6d.

73 See NA, MH 113/22.

74 Thorne Thorne, 'Results of the International Sanitary Conference of Rome', p. 138.

75 *Ibid.*

76 CLRO, *PSCP* (Jan. – June, 1885), letter from Collingridge to PSC, 23 March 1885.

77 CLRO, *PSCP* (Jan. – June, 1885), 'New Hospital – Gravesend – Medical Report, 11 June 1884' (my italics).

78 Baldwin, *Contagion and the State.*

79 E. Klein, *The Bacteria in Asiatic Cholera* (London: Macmillan, 1889), p. viii; also Klein and Gibbes, *An Inquiry into the Etiology of Asiatic Cholera* (London, 1885), p. 1.

80 See, Ogawa, 'Uneasy Bedfellows'; William Coleman, 'Koch's Comma Bacillus: The First Year', *Bulletin of the History of Medicine,* 61 (1987), 315–42; Evans, *Death in Hamburg,* pp. 265–71.

81 Harrison, *Public Health,* p. 112.

82 Klein, *The Bacteria in Asiatic Cholera,* pp. vii–viii.

83 Bruno Atalic, '1885 Cholera Controversy: Klein Versus Koch,' *Medical Humanities,* 36, 1 (2010), 43–7, p. 44.

84 Proceedings of a committee which assembled at the India Office ... for the purpose of considering a Report entitled 'An Inquiry into the Etiology of Asiatic Cholera', in Klein and Gibbes, *An Inquiry,* p. 15.

85 'The Official Refutation of Dr. Robert Koch's Theory of Cholera and Commas', *Quarterly Journal of Microscopical Science,* 26 (1886), 303–16; see also, Ogawa, 'Uneasy Bedfellows'.

86 'The Official Refutation', p. 316.

87 *Ibid.*

88 'Proc. Madras San. Comm'., no. 42, 1884, quoted in, Harrison, *Public Health,* p. 112.

89 *Report of the Quarantine Committee,* Royal College of Physicians, London [2248/2].

90 *Notes for the Quarantine Committee, May 1889,* Royal College of Physicians, London [2248/3]; for similar response see, Fayrer, 'The Origin, Habits and Diffusion of Cholera, and What May Be Bone to Prevent or Arrest Its Progress, and Mitigate Its Ravages' *Addresses and Papers, 1868–1888* (1886), p. 302, RAMC Collection (Wellcome Institute Library); and Sir J. Fayrer, *The Natural History and Epidemiology of Cholera–Being the Annual Oration of the Medical Society of London, May 7, 1888* (London: J & A Churchill, 1888), p. 32.

91 For further reading on these investigations see: Pelling, *Cholera, Fever and English Medicine*; Christopher Hamlin, 'Politics and Germ Theories in Victorian Britain: The Metropolitan Water Commissions of 1867–9 and 1892–3', in MacLeod (ed.), *Government and Expertise–Specialists, Administrators and Professionals, 1860–1919* (Cambridge: Cambridge University Press, 1988), pp. 110–27; Hamlin, *A Science of Impurity*; Anne Hardy, 'On the Cusp: Epidemiology and Bacteriology at the Local Government Board, 1890–1905', *Medical History* 42 (1998), pp. 328–46; Chapman, *Cholera Curable*; A.J. Wall, *Asiatic Cholera: Its History, Pathology, and Modern Treatment* (London: H.K. Lewis, 1893); Richard Thorne Thorne, *On the Progress of Preventive Medicine during the Victorian Era* (London: Shaw and Sons, 1988), Klein and Gibbes, *An Inquiry*; Isaacs, 'D.D. Cunningham'; Fayrer, *Natural History and Epidemiology of Cholera*.

92 Goodman, *International Health Organisations*; and Howard-Jones, 'The Scientific Background...', pp. 1–5.

3

1892

Even with the obstructive necessity of maintaining quarantine and the dual authority, the English System appeared to offer the perfect solution, both politically and economically, for the regulation of disease within the more porous borders of a Greater Britain. Ports were not closed spaces, separate from the towns and cities they served, but integrated urban, rural and riparian sanitation with ocean highways connecting Britain with its partners and possessions abroad. Quarantine, it seemed, had receded, an arcane law, maintained essentially in name only, almost completely unused and certainly unwanted.

Yet, in the final decade of the nineteenth century, only a few years before the repeal of the Quarantine Act, there was a short and intense period in which shipping companies and medical and sanitary officers rallied to demand that ships from certain Continental ports 'be quarantined.'[1] Port Medical Officers of Health sought to detain vessels for up to seven days and demanded various powers that had previously been possessed exclusively by the Quarantine Service. At the same time, the problems encountered in the maintenance of dual authority at the ports appeared to be worsening. The renewal of power to detain vessels was not, however, solicited by the Customs Service, but rather, was at the request of the Port Sanitary Authorities, who sought to harden the border and contract the space in and around the ports. The panic which led to this curious insistence on a renewal of strict quarantine procedures was the result of the cholera epidemic seen rapidly approaching Britain from the east in the summer of 1892.

Cholera on the move

The Western European and North American cholera epidemic of 1892 had, according to contemporary observers, two origins from whence it began its march westward.[2] The first was the outskirts of Paris, where the disease was identified in late March. It was believed to have been a recrudescence of former cholera epidemics in the area, which then extended down the Seine valley to the Le Havre by 5 July and northwards into Belgium by 20 July.[3] The second origin was in Asiatic Russia 'which ... received its infection as the result of an exceptional epidemic of cholera in British India during 1891; this being followed in the early months of 1892 by a recrudescence along the Indo-Afghan frontier.'[4] From Asiatic Russia the disease moved to European Russia where the first cases were said to have occurred in Astrakhan on 24 June, reaching St Petersburg on 1 August and Moscow on 5 August. It was in Poland before the end of the second week of August and at Hamburg, one of the busiest ports in the world, by 16 August. By the end of the month it had reached the United Kingdom, followed a couple of weeks later, in September, by its arrival in the United States.

What made this epidemic particularly alarming was the manner by which it appeared to spread across the Continent. Previous epidemics, such as the last major epidemic to attack Britain nearly thirty years earlier in 1866, primarily arrived with trade from Egypt and the Mediterranean. This time the progress of the epidemic across Europe was quickly associated with the westward migration of tens of thousands of Eastern European Jews fleeing persecution in Russia and the Pale of Settlement.[5] The disease was not arriving on board trading vessels, among crew and their small numbers of passengers, but in the massively overcrowded steerage holds of steamships. Although the epidemic of 1866 had arrived in Britain on trading vessels from Egypt and the Mediterranean, the source of the disease appeared sufficiently far removed; in 1892, those people who were believed to be responsible for importing the disease were congregating in ports on the western edge of Europe; some, having made the crossing to Britain, remained and settled within the country.[6] The disease was on the doorstep. The transportation of thousands of migrants from Russia, west through Europe and ultimately, for most migrants, to the United States, was big business, quickly and on the whole efficiently operated. It was the numbers and speed with which the migrations appeared to move across Europe as well as the accompanying prejudices associated with the cultural, religious and physical difference of the migrants which was particularly frightening to contemporary observers of the 1892 epidemic.

The migration principally began in 1881 when the assassination of Tsar Alexander II ignited a wave of anti-Semitic retaliatory pogroms against Jews across Russia and the Pale. One of the Tsar's assassins had been Jewish – reason enough to provoke violence where prejudice already existed. Unrecorded numbers were killed, thousands injured, and Jewish property suffered hundreds of thousands of pounds worth of damage. Following the violence, only months after the widespread devastation of the pogroms, the new Tsar introduced legislation which severely restricted the liberty of Jews. The so-called Temporary Laws (although they remained in place for over thirty years) forbade Jews to live outside designated towns within the Pale, to purchase property, to access secondary or higher education or to vote. The Jewish community was forced to submit a far greater proportion of its population to extended military service, during which only the lowest ranks of the army were available and promotion or advancement was impossible.[7] These conditions and numerous other anti-Semitic laws and pogroms continued over the following decades and encouraged many who were subsequently constrained or persecuted to seek refuge in the reputedly more liberal west. Some settled in Western Europe and Great Britain, although most – almost half a million by 1892[8] – migrated to the United States. Those en route to America, when travelling through Europe and Britain, were termed 'transmigrants'.

Although Eastern European migration continued on a large scale through the 1880s until around 1914, 1892 and 1893 were particularly busy years. The social, political and religious persecution suffered by Russian Jews since the beginning of the 1880s was compounded from 1891–92 by severe famine and by a new, and especially rampant, epidemic of cholera which in the summer of 1892 claimed an estimated 300,000 lives in Russia and affected a total of around 620,000 people.[9] Limited access for Jews to medical services in Russia and the potency of peasant superstitions about the illness and the medical profession meant that public health efforts were generally ineffectual and the disease spread with frightening rapidity.[10] Thus, the number of people fleeing Russia increased significantly, as riots and panic escalated. Emigrants headed West both to settle in the more liberal regimes of Western nations and to escape the 'degrading violence' of one of the most dreaded diseases of the nineteenth century.[11]

However, despite the migrants' attempts to flee infection, cholera moved west with them, following the routes they travelled en route to America. The principal routes were west from Russia and the Pale, through Germany to Dutch, Belgian or German ports, or from Baltic ports, particularly Libau (Liepāja in western Latvia). The busiest migrant – and trade – port in Europe was Hamburg, and it was there that cholera had its most devastating effect in Western Europe. The first case occurred in a sewerage worker on 14 August, who died the following day. Each successive day saw the disease extend to more and more people. Two new cases were reported on the 16th, four on the 17th, twelve on the 18th and thirty-one by the 19th.[12] From one of the cases on 17 August, a sample was taken for bacteriological testing, but the tests did not produce a pure culture of comma bacillus until the 22nd, meaning that clinical observation continued to be the primary means of diagnosis. The Imperial Government in Berlin was informed on 23 August and by 26 August the number of newly reported cases occurring in the city that day had reached one thousand.[13] Yet, officials did not announce to the world that Hamburg was an infected port until 26 August 1892. Anxious to rid the busy port of the rapidly increasing and expensive number of migrants accumulating in the city, the President of the Hamburg Medical Board, Senator Gerhard Hachmann, and his colleagues withheld the information and allowed the departure of a number of infected ships bound for America,[14] primarily because once domestic and foreign quarantines were imposed on the city, the emigrants stranded in Hamburg would become the financial burden of the Hamburg Senate. In all, three over-crowded Hamburg–America Line ships departed from the infected port with clean Bills of Health between 17 and 25 August for direct passage to New York, the second largest port in the world. The first ship to arrive there carrying the cholera bacillus was the *SS Moravia*. Prior to its departure on the 17th Hachmann had assured the American Vice-Consul in Hamburg that no cholera was present in the city and the steamship departed with a clean Bill of Health.

Although the Imperial Government did not officially announce the presence of cholera until 26 August, the British Consulate in Hamburg telegraphed London on 25 August stating that the disease was present in the port. But by then cholera had already crossed the North Sea. The first case appeared in Grangemouth on the East Coast of Scotland on 19 August. On 25 August a vessel carrying Russian Jewish transmigrants from Hamburg arrived in Leith. They boarded a train to Glasgow, where they were to pick up the boat to America, and it was there that two of the passengers began to display some of the symptoms of cholera: 'The patients, when received into Belvidere,[15] had the cold extremities, the livid fingers and toes, the stricken expression, the sighing hollow voice and the profound prostration so characteristic of true cholera'.[16] In London a vessel carrying three fatal cases of cholera, all Russian Jewish emigrants en route to America from Hamburg, arrived on 25 August, having sailed from Hamburg after it was known that cholera was present in the city but before it was officially announced. In Liverpool, on 29 August, three cases of cholera were identified among a group of immigrants who had arrived by train from the eastern English port of Hull.

British sanitary officials had been making preparations for the imminent arrival of cholera well before the disease arrived in Hamburg or appeared in British ports. As Richard Thorne Thorne, now Chief Medical Officer to the Local Government Board, wrote in the *Annual Report of the Local Government Board, 1892*, the spread of the disease into Western Europe was, from the beginning of the summer, expected to accompany Eastern European migrants:

> And, when the disease was evidently about to invade those provinces of Russia which are within the Pale of Settlement for the Jews, and from which emigration of Russian Jews across Germany and thence to this country was at the time in rapid and continual progress, it became necessary at once to warn the authorities of those English Ports at which these immigrants and trans-migrants were landing.[17]

Considering the devastation which the 1892 epidemic caused in parts of Europe, America, the Middle East, as well as Northern Africa, British precautions proved comparably effective. St Petersburg and Hamburg, for example, suffered thousands of deaths in late August and early September 1892, while the *British Medical Journal* was able to report confidently that only twenty-four cases of undoubted cholera were reported in England and Wales in the same period.[18] Nevertheless, British sanitary officers remained poised, defences in place, alert to the possible danger – seen as emanating directly from the tens of thousands of Eastern European migrants who had uprooted from family, friends and home in the summer of that year, as they fled disease and persecution in Russia.

Their anticipated arrival – frequently characterised as an 'invasion' – was awaited with growing concern and the mobilisation of all the apposite military rhetoric:

> From the first appearance of the cloud not bigger than a man's hand in the East, the march of the disease was carefully watched from Whitehall, and as soon as it was seen to be approaching the provinces in Russia within the pale of settlement from which the

emigration of Jews is constantly taking place into and across this country, inspectors were sent by the Local Government Board to all the ports on the east coast to warn the local authorities of the probable advent of cholera, and to urge them to complete their sanitary defences in time to repel the threatened invasion ... The danger was in the present instance greatly aggravated by the character of the people conveying the infection ... There is reason to believe that the enemy has been successfully repulsed for the time, but it is important to realise that the danger is not yet over.[19]

From the beginning, Eastern European emigrants were seen as 'the chief source of danger',[20] reconfirming the notion that cholera was essentially a 'foreign disease'.[21]

Paul Weindling has disputed the claim that Jews were responsible for the spread of cholera from Eastern to Western Europe and North America. He claims that 'given that transmigrants did not "cause" cholera in other port cities, notably Bremen, to accept that Russian Jews had to be the primary cause and carriers of cholera would be to swallow the anti-Semitic prejudices of the time'.[22] He argues that the assumption made by scholars such as Richard Evans that cholera was brought to Hamburg and subsequently west by *Ostjuden*, was more a case of 'conjecture rather than epidemiologically proven'.[23] Despite widespread belief among the authorities in Hamburg that the transmigrants were responsible for the outbreak of the epidemic, Weindling insists that 'such prejudices did not infect expert opinion',[24] – i.e. Koch's. Rather, Koch's expertise and scientific reasoning allowed him to transcend any anti-Semitism present in Hamburg during the epidemic and recognise that cholera had spread because of the failure of the Hamburg authorities to disinfect the waste water from the migrants' lodgings at the port.[25]

Whether or not the failure to maintain sanitary conditions at the ports was the actual reason why cholera was transmitted so extensively throughout the city, however, is irrelevant. Overwhelmingly, contemporaries in both Europe (including Britain) and America blamed Jewish migrants for the disease, and much of the fear which existed in relation to the 1892 epidemic was a direct reflection of this. Retrospectively, Weindling may be perfectly correct in stating that epidemiologically Eastern European Jews did not deserve the accusation that they, particularly, spread the disease. The value of his analysis lies in clarifying the anti-Semitic nature of much of the response in Hamburg and other infected ports to the transmigrants as disease carriers.[26] But, as Weindling himself states, 'the view held at the time' was that 'Russian Jews caused the Hamburg cholera epidemic', as well as the New York epidemic and the introduction of cholera into the Port of London. What is important is not the legitimacy of contemporary fears and accusations, but how they affected popular perceptions in 1892, the implementation of policy and medical practice, and the contemporary texts through which we can observe these processes.

For decades, British public health officials had begun to feel secure behind the preventive space constructed at the ports. The Port Sanitary Authorities, in cooperation with local sanitary authorities, the entire infrastructure of sanitation, as well as the Customs Service, had overwhelming public and government support in its ability to provide the necessary precautions against any threatened invasion of imported infectious disease. The Prime Minister, Robert Gascoyne-Cecil, Marquess of Salisbury, wrote to Thorne Thorne in May 1892, while the disease was still at a 'safe' distance, conveying the confidence maintained in the English System:

> There has always been, as you are aware, a considerable divergence of views between the teachings put forward by the medical authorities and accepted by public opinion in England and in India, and that which has prevailed upon the Continent, as to the efficacy of quarantine as a safeguard against the contagion of cholera and some other diseases. The tendency of English opinion has been rather to look to measures of sanitary improvement as the best prophylactic against cholera ...[27]

However, in the summer of 1892 the almost complacent attitude which had developed toward diseases such as cholera[28] was replaced by quite visible anxiety among public health officials, as they saw the disease advance into Western Europe. The comfortable confidence in the English System which had accompanied British delegates to the International Sanitary Conferences and allowed for such assured defiance of quarantine, was suddenly forgotten, and for a time, even the most confident sometimes 'had trouble holding their nerve'.[29] *The Lancet*, which had exhibited seemingly stalwart support for sanitary surveillance at the ports, was among those to flinch:

> It has been assumed by some sanitary authorities that the mere fact of our system of 'medical inspection' exhibiting certain interstices through which cholera might creep was sufficient to warrant them in crying out for a return to quarantine restrictions, some wishing

that all vessels from infected places should be kept in detention two days, others three and four days, and others five days. As to this demand, we would ... point out that the English System never laid claim to any infallible pretensions to keep cholera altogether out of the country.[30]

What caused this change of heart and waning of confidence? Despite what Weindling argues, and the obvious anti-Semitism of the time, it had much to do with the fact that the perceived source of the disease was the often 'bedraggled', 'exotic' looking Eastern European Jews, arriving in their thousands at ports as immigrants or transmigrants continuing on to a final destination in America or elsewhere. Indeed, much of the fear and panic of 1892 was due, in part, to the fact that for many contemporaries, these migrants embodied a physical difference and 'exoticness' which enabled easy association with the notoriously 'exotic' disease. Such a characterisation enabled any other fears associated with their arrival to be easily projected onto their supposed role as cholera carriers. Their 'foreignness' and the 'foreignness' of cholera appeared to be one and the same.

This assumed correlation implied a reversion to old ideas about contagion or an acceptance of the bacteriological concept of cholera transmission. However, the idea that the migrants could bring disease with them was easily accommodated into existing medical theories about port health, which still resisted Koch's bacillus. As an article in *The Lancet* explained, the migrants did not import the disease through any process of contagion, as was articulated in bacteriological models of cholera aetiology, but rather were seen within a Pettenkofean model of disease; they brought with them the 'locality' within which disease could generate:

A number of immigrants arriving from an infected district – possibly dirty as regards their persons, and still more so as regards their clothes – may be provisionally regarded as so many *minute migratory fragments of the locality whence they came.*[31]

Although somewhat extreme, this example demonstrates the significant place Pettenkofean theories still occupied in British aetiological thought when it came to disease at the ports. These theories were gradated between the extreme localism demonstrated above, and the bacteriological notion that 'if it be true that the disease is caused by a living organism, whatever it may be, it is certain that the organism goes out in the bowel discharges of the patient.'[32] Both ways, 'it [was] not cholera so much that [had] to be feared, it [was] rather the filth which may serve as a breeding-ground for imported infections'.[33] Invariably, migrants and transmigrants were described and prefaced with the word 'filthy'. During 1892 the use of the word 'filth' with regard to cholera was often closely associated with steerage-class migrants – 'the very class that might be picked out as most likely to spread the disease'.[34]

So, migrants brought 'filthy' and thus diseased space within the controlled environment of the 'English' sanitary zone. What thus needed to be targeted in devising prophylactic strategies at the ports in 1892 was this 'filth' and these 'migrating localities' of disease – the Eastern European immigrants and transmigrants. Weindling might argue that this is 'swallowing the anti-Semitic prejudices of the time', but in order to understand the particular and additional preventive measures put in place during 1892, and the subsequent effects the epidemic had on British port health, it is necessary to acknowledge the strength of these contemporary fears.

It is not surprising then that the primary precautions put in place to avoid the importation of cholera in 1892 were directed particularly toward the migrants, as well as surveillance continuing for the arrival of general port traffic. The General Cholera Order, issued by the Local Government Board on 6 September 1892, was the primary instrument for the control of cholera cases, and it built on the powers of the previous Cholera Order of 28 August 1890. The latter required Customs boarding officers to identify cases of the disease and then report them to the Port Sanitary Authorities. With the increased danger posed by the 1892 epidemic, however, the Local Government Board altered the old Order and introduced the authority, in London at least, for a Medical Officer of the Port Sanitary Authority to visit every ship which arrived into the port, accompanying the Officers of Customs.

Under the Quarantine Act, a Medical Officer of Health who boarded a vessel before the Quarantine Officer had arrived to undertake his own inspection was forbidden to leave the ship until granted a formal Quarantine clearance by an officer of the Customs Service.[35] The Act clearly stated that anyone who 'quit' a quarantinable vessel would be liable to up to six months imprisonment or a fine of three hundred pounds.[36] Every vessel suspected of being infected with cholera thus came initially within the governance of the Quarantine Act until formally cleared and passed over to the Port Sanitary Authority. By boarding vessels with the Quarantine Officer, as the 1892 Order allowed, a Medical Officer could be granted clearance on the spot and could thus continue with his own inspection without restriction.[37]

Focussing more specifically on the arrival of migrants into London were Articles 2 and 3 of the 1892 Cholera Order. They denied any passenger permission to land who could not provide a 'correct' address in the city or show means of supporting themselves.[38] Although Medical Officers of Health had previously obtained addresses when they inspected infected or suspected ships and forwarded these to local sanitary authorities, the new Order went further by preventing the landing of those passengers whose lodging could not be fully verified. This was expressly targeted toward migrants, as the Local Government Board made clear in the following report on the Cholera Regulations:

> ...it appears that large numbers of aliens in a filthy and otherwise unwholesome condition are now being brought into this country, and that the danger of the introduction of cholera is thereby increased. Under these circumstances the board have thought it desirable to issue an order altering the Cholera regulations ... so as to impose certain restrictions on the landing of persons from ships bringing passengers of the class referred to ...[39]

Those immigrants whose addresses could not be verified were 'returned in the ship,'[40] and the masters of vessels who landed passengers who had not been discharged by a Medical Officer could be fined up to £50. Surveillance was key to the English System; without it the integrity and security of the sanitary zone could not function. The integrated space of the port, the city and the sea was severed with the act of unauthorised and unsupervised 'landing'. The land detached from the sea and the defined spaces of 'inside' and 'outside' came back into sharp relief. That those people who were landing – and the disease with which they were associated – embodied the 'outside' only intensified the rupture. So, while the English System under ordinary circumstances required only the gathering and sharing of information among sanitary authorities to assimilate 'outside' and 'inside' space, the new Cholera Order evaluated 'inside' space as being appropriate or not for the integration of a particular type of 'outside' space exemplified by the body of the immigrant.

To achieve this, intended addresses of immigrants were verified against a list of registered lodging houses to establish whether the address existed. This was necessary, a 'careful investigation' informed the Local Government Board, because 'there is difficulty ... dealing with the Jewish immigrants', and that 'about 25 or 30% of the addresses given are untrustworthy'.[41] Addresses were also checked against a list of lodging houses recorded as 'unsanitary'. These checks, although primarily concerned with the residences of 'Jewish immigrants', were applied to all steerage-class passengers. The German Young Men's Christian Association complained formally to the Port Sanitary Committee when they discovered they had been placed on the 'unsanitary lodging house' list:

> The Medical Man, who has the charge of calling on the steamboats on their arrival in London coming from the Continent (Hamburg and Rotterdam) in order to make sure if the passengers are in good health and to find out to what Hotel or private house they intend to go, has on several occasions (which have come to our notice) forbidden that passengers should come to our Hotel at the above address [Finsbury Sq., London] saying that the sanitary condition of it does not give satisfaction.[42]

The German YMCA, which had three 'hotels' in London, was unaware that their property had been placed on the 'unsanitary' list. Their complaints were an attempt to gain some compensation for the losses incurred, to have the property removed from the list, and to disassociate themselves from any injurious connection with Eastern European immigrants. The Assistant Medical Officer was quoted as remarking 'I'm afraid, Captain, that Hotel is on my black list' – referring to a page in his pocket-book. Collingridge claimed that no instructions regarding the hotel had ever been given to the Medical Officers. Instead, he explained 'all that this implies either is that there is some doubt as to the passengers themselves or that there is some difficulty in verifying the address'.[43] A solicitor representing the German YMCA investigated the case and interviewed a number of masters of vessels and passengers. These testimonies provide a valuable and rare insight into how the inspections were carried out:

> All the passengers were summoned to the Cabin and I was the first who arrived. In the Cabin were the Captain, the Doctor, a Policeman, and the ship's Steward. I understand English sufficiently to know what is being said but I do not speak it well. The Captain's name was Brocsen (who acted as interpreter between the Dr., who spoke English, and the passengers who spoke German). The Captain presented to the Dr. a list of all the passengers with the address of their proposed destinations, reading my name with 28 Finsbury Square as my proposed address. This address did not appear to be satisfactory to the Dr. but the Captain urged very strongly that the address was quite suitable and the Dr. asked me thro' the Captain

> from whom I got the address and I replied, from a similar home in
> Hamburg. The Dr. shrugged his shoulders and said I can't pass your
> address, but gave no reason. He said tomorrow another Dr. will
> come and give you a final decision.[44]

The man was eventually granted permission to land,[45] but not all migrants were so fortunate. In October 1892, for instance, four vessels which arrived in London carrying European migrants were forced to return to the Continent with a number of unfortunate people still aboard.[46]

Throughout 1892–93 the *British Medical Journal* printed extensive articles and reports about the progress of the cholera epidemic, on treatment, and increasingly on the constant potential of the disease's importation into Britain via the 'huge' stream of Eastern Europeans and other steerage-class migrants. Concern was met with occasional assurance, as the Medical Officer of Health for the Whitechapel District reported in September: 'although inhabited by many foreigners of the alien class, this district has been altogether free from cholera. The doubtful cases which were landed from Hamburg, and attended to in the London Hospital, proved to be severe enteritis.'[47] However, during the anticipated crisis of 1892–93, most attention directed toward European immigrants was negative and provocative. Information had been gathered during previous epidemics relating to infected and suspected ports throughout the world but generally had not targeted one place or population over another. In 1892–93, the source of the epidemic was almost exclusively directed toward migrants. Unlike the infected or suspected foreign ports which were monitored in previous epidemics and which lay beyond the reach of sanitary precautions, 'filthy' migrants penetrated the orderly composition of the English System. They entered into the carefully managed space created by the sanitary zone, injecting into it 'foreign' localities in their 'foreign' bodies. Controlling how and where the migrants inhabited 'domestic' space sought to restore order to the system, assimilating them within the now greatly contracted borders of the sanitary zone.

Observation

The treatment of the steamship *Gemma*, which I discussed in the introduction to this book, was in many ways typical of the general process of prevention that operated in the Port of London in 1892.

Yet in many ways it marked a pivotal shift in the particular focus and classification of disease that had guided the operation of the English System from its inception. The 'filthy' *Gemma* migrants came to represent as much a category of risk as the 'exotic' disease cholera, and their treatment reflects the transition that began to occur in 1892 from a concentration, in the management of public health at the ports, from the imported disease to the particular 'nature' of those who imported it.

When the *Gemma* arrived at Gravesend on 25 August, the attending Customs Boarding Officer determined that there was illness on board. Unable to contact the Quarantine Medical Officer, which was normal procedure, he contacted the Acting Port Medical Officer of Health for Gravesend, Dr Philip Whitcombe. Whitcombe examined the passengers and concluded that they were infected with 'Asiatic' cholera. He was shortly joined by Collingridge who was able to confirm the diagnosis. Complying with the Quarantine Act, Customs then gave clearance for the vessel to be released into the care of the Port Sanitary Authority. The crew, first- and second-class passengers were permitted to disembark after a rudimentary inspection and once their intended accommodations in the city had been recorded. The three infected immigrants were removed to the Port Sanitary Isolation Hospital at Denton, along with all of their bedding and personal effects, which were subsequently burned. The third-class immigrant passengers remained on board the *Gemma*. On the 25th, Collingridge and his colleagues 'set to work', cleaning the 'filthiness' from their bodies and belongings, and enquiries were made for finding a 'spare ship' for their accommodation 'until they could supply him with satisfactory statements as to their future addresses in London'.[48] However, as an appropriate vessel could not be found, it was decided that they could be accommodated in tents on 'a spare couple of acres' at the Port Sanitary Hospital site.[49] There they remained until 31 August when they were all released under close surveillance of the local sanitary authorities. Nevertheless, some of the migrants travelled on to Manchester without the knowledge of the Local Government Board, who were only informed the next day that three had been 'found' in Manchester. All were in 'good health'. Responding to the presence of the *Gemma* migrants in the city, the Manchester sanitary authorities 'passed a series of resolutions by a special meeting of our hospital committee', including the immediate publication 'of a handbill of sanitary precautions against cholera and choleraic diarrhoea, printed in Hebrew, together with a translation in English language'.[50]

The case of the *Gemma* raises a number of interesting and illuminating points. Firstly, even as late as the 1892 epidemic, cholera was still deemed to be a 'quarantinable' disease, and thus not yet fully incorporated into the sanitary system. The Customs Officer who, as in usual practice, was the first boarding authority, was required to contact the Quarantine Medical Officer. He being unobtainable, his *second* choice had been to contact the Port Medical Officer. It was only once the Customs Authority provided clearance that the Port Sanitary Authority were able to assume responsibility for 'care' of the ship and its passengers.

Secondly, both Whitcombe and Collingridge made their official diagnoses of cholera without bacteriological testing. While diagnostic testing for the disease was carried out in laboratories during the epidemic in Germany and the United States for example, clinical diagnoses only were used in Britain's ports. Koch's bacteriological cause of cholera, which had been so roundly rejected at the 1885 International Sanitary Conference, still had not been integrated into the management of the disease at the ports. Indeed, bacteriological testing for cholera at the ports did not appear until late 1894, when Klein confirmed the presence of cholera in the post-mortem examination of a sailor who had arrived on the steamship *Balmore*. The examination showed 'in microscopic specimen and cultivation typical cholera'.[51] Even then, bacteriological confirmation only arrived at the Local Government Board nine days after the *Balmore* had sailed into the Port of London from St. Petersburg. The six other sailors who displayed symptoms of the disease were immediately removed to Denton on arrival into London; the other passengers and crew had been released into the community under the surveillance of local Medical Officers. Specimens were also taken from them, which confirmed cholera, although by the time the results were received by Thorne Thorne, four were dead and the remaining two were convalescing.

In 1892 Medical Officers still relied primarily on clinical judgement in determining cases of cholera. Diagnosis by observable symptoms was clearly demonstrated in notes of the cholera cases which arrived in Glasgow's Belvidere Infectious Diseases Hospital in late August 1892. The Superintendent of the Hospital, Dr. James Allan, published his case notes in *The Lancet* on 2 September:

> There are at present two cholera cases in Belvidere. The patients (a man and a woman) are Russian (Jew) emigrants, who reached Glasgow by Hamburg and Leith. The male patient was admitted to

hospital at 1 o'clock on the morning of the 27ᵗʰ ult... *The patient's appearance was a confirmation of the diagnosis (cholera).* The pinched face, cold, dark, shrunken hands, which were feebly tossed about, and the husky moaning voice conveyed a sufficiently dismal impression.[52]

Finally, Whitcombe remarked in his report of the *Gemma* that 'the ship was placed in quarantine'.[53] In many ways, the detention of its migrants resembled quarantine more than it did the English System, which professed only to incarcerate those people who displayed symptoms of disease, and it is noteworthy that Whitcombe made this distinction even if only through the terminology he chose to employ. However, despite usual widespread opposition to quarantine, the period of detention imposed on the *Gemma* migrants was widely supported. An article in *The Lancet* in October 1892 acknowledged that

> This ... action went beyond the powers actually conferred under the Cholera Order ... but the judicious action taken in this matter ... received its justification a few days later when an additional order was issued to meet the case of *such passengers as these* – that is to say, of persons whom it is impossible to keep under observation on arrival from an infected place or infected vessel, for the simple reason that they have no home or destination. Dr Collingridge's action at the time received full public support ...[54]

As in the response elicited from Collingridge and his colleagues, the central problem here was seen to lie in 'such passengers as these' rather than in the disease itself. An undercurrent of unease was exposed, revealing a lack of total confidence, even among Medical Officers, in the ability of the system to deal with the particular 'category' of disease embodied by the migrants. By insisting on the detention of the *Gemma* migrants at the port, Collingridge revealed a level of distrust in the English System, either with regard to the safety net of surveillance, or the local sanitary environment, or both. He clearly was not willing to release the migrants before the expiration of a short incubation period. Despite the continued rhetoric which rejected quarantine, the anxiety about the particular 'migrating locations' of disease, represented in the bodies and 'foreignness' of the migrants in the summer of 1892, could not be allayed by the operation of sanitary systems alone. In public lectures and publications, both before and after 1892, Collingridge declared his opposition to the principles of quarantine and imposed detention. Yet, during that summer he wrote to the Port Sanitary

Committee on a number of occasions about his frustration at being unable to isolate and detain immigrant vessels.[55]

The three passengers on the *Gemma* who displayed symptoms of the disease could easily be removed to the isolation hospital at Denton. However, the only recourse available to Collingridge to keep the other immigrants detained for further observation was to insist that the information they supplied about their addresses in London was unreliable. Collingridge was unwilling to entrust the *Gemma* migrants to the local authorities, as was customary, but rather insisted that they remain under his supervision at the port. On 25 August, as the vessel arrived into London, Collingridge had telegraphed Hugh Owen, Secretary to the Local Government Board, informing him of his plans for the *Gemma* migrants: 'Gemma from Hamburg arrived three cases cholera on board have taken these to port hospital will fumigate effects and detain emigrants for observation.'[56]

The legitimacy of the addresses supplied by the steerage passengers was inconsequential since the decision to detain them had already been made before any inspection had taken place. Surprisingly, Owen replied with hearty support for the idea:

> When emigrants leave ship most important that they should be kept together and under observation. Could not port sanitary authority utilise some building or make other provision for this, meantime emigrants should be detained on ship as long as circumstances permit.[57]

Indeed, as *The Times* reported, while being careful to note that any extension of the period of detention for healthy passengers was *not* a return to quarantine procedures, the circumstances of 1892 appeared to require a prolongation of the present period and method of observation for healthy passengers 'if they arrive in suspicious circumstances ...'[58]

These 'suspicious circumstances', clearly a euphemism for steerage-class migrants, required additional measures to protect against the particular type of threat they posed. Ordinary observation for monitoring disease, whatever its origin, within the controlled space of domestic sanitary management, would not be able to integrate the 'foreign' environment introduced by this class of migrants, whether they settled in the city or were merely temporarily housed in one of its many lodging houses. Their bodies and the localities they inhabited trespassed upon the neatly enumerated, ordered and monitored sanitary system that had integrated the ports and maritime space into the domestic sanitary environment and had pushed its 'virtues' beyond the littoral, creating the sanitary zone and defining it as particularly 'English'. The neatness of the English System in its present form did not account for 'such passengers as these', and once the crisis was over there would need to be some reassessment of the capabilities and priorities of Britain's port health system.

The impact of 1892

The 1892 cholera epidemic has consistently been overlooked – with the notable exception of Richard Evans' classic work on Hamburg – and is rarely considered to have been of any consequence in the British Isles. However, its importance in effecting change in the management of port health was significant and was certainly recognized by contemporaries. The *New York Medical Journal* captured the moment of change in an article published just as the epidemic started to recede:

> CHOLERA A POSSIBLE BLESSING IN DISGUISE
> Dr Collingridge, of the Port of London, is one of those men who can discern a 'silver lining' to even the dark cloud of epidemic cholera. He is reported in one of the London papers to have said, in substance: In fact the cholera is *the best thing* that can happen to us. If we did not get a scare about once in three years, our sanitation would soon get neglected. Cholera passed our first great Public Health Act. It formed our port sanitary regulations and authority. These acts have saved more human lives than ever cholera destroyed since the world began. If the cholera experience of the Port of New York in 1892 can do for us something intelligent, humane, or even human, in the way of sanitary legislation, these squalid immigrants, who have excited so much harsh comment, may prove to be angels in disguise to 'a plenitude of generations yet to come'.[59]

The immediate aftermath of the epidemic brought reflection about the respective roles of the Port Sanitary Authorities and Quarantine Service. Quickly forgetting their initial, and sometimes continued, regression into quarantinist thinking, those at the forefront of the English System emerged from 1892 full of confidence. The Local Government Board began to insist on the permanent transferral of many of the powers the Port Sanitary Authorities had temporarily been issued with during the epidemic, while the role of quarantine in British ports was again thrown into question.

Having experienced no real threat of a large-scale cholera epidemic since the Public Health Act of 1872, the Port Sanitary Authorities had previously not had any opportunity to prove the effectiveness of the system with regard to cholera. As cholera was a primary factor in the establishment of the English System and this system had been defended by Britain at the International Sanitary Conferences as the only viable alternative to the antiquated system of quarantine, the 1892 epidemic served as a critical test case. And, the results were overwhelming. While quarantined Hamburg reported almost 17,000 cases, in Britain no cases of cholera extended beyond the thirty-five infected individuals who arrived at ports from abroad. With this evident affirmation of the efficacy of sanitary practice over quarantine, the Port Sanitary Authorities and Local Government Board began asserting their control over the ports.

A week before Christmas, the jubilant Port Sanitary Committee convened a conference in London with the purpose of reviewing the management of that summer's epidemic, how preparations might best be made for the next epidemic anticipated in the following year, and how the capacities of the sanitary authorities might be strengthened and consolidated.[60] It was attended by 122 delegates from forty-two Port Sanitary Authorities around England and Wales, including Port Medical Officers of Health, Medical Officers of Health, Port Sanitary Authority Chairmen, Mayors, Inspectors of Nuisances and Town Clerks.[61]

One of the first orders of business reiterated and reinforced the fundamental priority that had undergirded all discussions of maritime disease control throughout the second half of the century. It was essential that trading vessels and their goods were processed and allowed to proceed with a minimum of interference. As such, all agreed that during crises such as 1892, inspections should continue throughout the night in large ports such as London, even if it required the appointment of additional staff. These men would inspect all trading vessels, while those 'vessels carrying emigrants requiring special inspection, requiring an inspection for an hour, or an hour and a half' should always be visited last in order to 'prevent vexatious delays and expensive detention of the [other] vessels at the cost of shipowners'.[62] So, the open fluidity of the ports would be maintained for trading vessels, but migrant vessels would be treated differently, having longer inspections and greater waiting periods.

The importance of category making, which had become such an essential component in international disease control efforts, as exemplified at the sanitary conferences, was applied at all levels of discussion and was critical to the way members of the conference began to reconstitute the sanitary zone. Ships were categorized as involved in either commerce or migration, either integrated into the English System or pushed to its margins. The classification of foreign ports was also fundamental in drawing the boundaries of the sanitary zone. Inspection and surveillance, which underpinned the system and space it defined relied on information about the location of infection. Delegates at the meeting agreed that the classification and identification of 'infected' ports was key to their work. In order to inspect every vessel that had sailed from an infected port it was necessary to accurately identify which ports were 'infected' and subsequently when they were declared 'free of infection'. However, as Henry Armstrong, the Port Medical Officer for Newcastle-upon-Tyne noted, designating and compiling appropriate categories for foreign ports was no simple task:

> The meaning of the word 'infected' at present is not defined at all. It stands alone and is the only word used in cholera regulations. ... There is no provision for 'suspected'; therefore, anyone interpreting 'infected' must interpret it to mean either known to be infected or suspected of being infected.[63]

So, although the delegates deemed it necessary to issue the Port Sanitary Authorities with an official list of 'infected' ports, the practical realities of obtaining such data were problematic. If information about the presence of disease in a port were to emanate from British Consuls (assuming they were informed of the presence of cholera in their port), it would take too long to reach all the port and regional authorities for it to be of any use. Furthermore, and more importantly, the possible implications any such *official* list would have for trade would be too detrimental. As Collingridge explained to the conference,

> an official list published by the Local Government Board is theoretical and imaginary. It is impossible to carry it out. No government could undertake it, and no government would undertake it. At present the whole of the littoral from St Petersburg to Lorient is infected with cholera. If any Government Department issued a notice that all those ports are infected, where should we be with regard to British commerce? Hamburg is officially declared free from Cholera, but there are cases of Cholera from Hamburg now. If you are to have a list of infected ports – and such a list is desirable for

our own purposes – it must be issued on our own responsibility, because the Government would not, and could not, declare Hamburg to be infected at the present moment, although everybody knows that it is.[64]

Thus the delegates agreed that, rather than having to rely upon 'newspaper reports',[65] the Port Sanitary Authority of London would issue its own *unofficial* list, categorizing foreign ports, which would be forwarded to the other authorities. As such there would be a uniform 'private list of "dangerous" ports – you may keep out the word "infected"'.[66]

Another essential category related to migrants. The conference marked a pivotal transition in thinking about disease control practices at the ports particularly for those ships which arrived from infected ports carrying steerage-class migrants. Categorised separately from 'ordinary' trading vessels, these ships were deemed to require special sanitary attention. Part of the issue, as it was constructed by the sanitary authorities, was that once a vessel had been granted quarantine clearance by Customs (if there was, and had been, no case of cholera on board during the voyage) it was free to proceed into the port. As the Customs Service was the only authority with the power to detain vessels, without a Quarantine Officer being present Port Medical Officers could not prevent migrant vessels, arriving from 'infected' ports, from coming up to the docks. In addition, if the Medical Officer was engaged elsewhere there was no way to hold these vessels until someone became available to carry out the inspection. Consequently, there was no opportunity to deter potentially diseased migrants from disembarking, and the names and addresses of those on board would go unrecorded. The crucial surveillance of the sanitary system would be lost.

The Medical Officers at the conference therefore proposed unanimously that extra power should be conferred upon them if they were to continue to protect the ports from the particular risk of cholera imported by migrants. The ability to detain a vessel lay solely with the Customs Officers acting under the Quarantine Act. Undermining the 'Quarantine Certificate', the delegates claimed that quarantine clearance to enter the docks was 'given as a mere matter of form, and was therefore useless'.[67] As such, it was agreed that a proposal should be put to the Local Government Board to imbue the Port Sanitary Authorities with the power to impose a period of detention of six hours, three hours before inspection and three hours afterward, for all vessels sailing from ports falling within their category of 'infected'. It was argued that clearance should be issued by a Medical Officer of Health, rather than a Customs Officer, after he had made his own, more informed, examination. Similarly, the Port Sanitary Authorities should be granted the authority to penalise anyone who provided false answers during an inspection.

Overwhelmingly, the goal of the conference seemed to be to finally reallocate arbitration of the geo-border away from the old quarantine and Customs Service to the new English System. As Collingridge, in his role as Chairman, elucidated:

> What we are doing here is gradually to remove the present quarantine powers. Everything suggested today is in the direction of removing the onus of medical inspection from the Customs to the Port Sanitary Authority – a most desirable change.[68]

The Port Sanitary Authorities of Scotland did not attend the conference in London. While almost identical to the English and Welsh authorities, the Scottish Port Sanitary Authorities had been established under the separate Public Health (Scotland) Acts. No similar conference, following the 1892 epidemic, was convened in Scotland. One reason for this was that the dual authority of Customs and Port Sanitary Authority did not appear, in Glasgow and Greenock at least, to have created the same problems as were encountered elsewhere. Of course, the same difficulties arose with regard to jurisdictional boundaries, yet the issues relating to detention and notification were more satisfactorily attended to in Scotland, particularly immediately after the 1892 crisis. An Order in Council of 1893 conferred greater powers on both the Customs Service and the Port Sanitary Authorities of Scotland than was available to corresponding officers in England and Wales.[69] This enabled the Scottish Port Sanitary Authorities greater power in classifying which vessels ought to be detained by Customs for their own inspections.[70] Any vessel, therefore, which arrived in a Scottish port from a port which the Medical Officers of Health deemed to be infected with cholera, could be detained by Officers of the Customs Service until the Medical Officer was informed and brought to the ship.[71] Even if the vessel held a Clean Bill of Health, issued at the port of departure, the fact that the ship departed from a port which the Scottish Medical Officers deemed 'infectious' was sufficient for Customs to detain it.[72]

Although a level of cooperation was reached between the two authorities in Scotland, this was not the case in England and Wales, and the London conference of Port Medical Officers became the setting for the beginning of cautious proceedings aimed at the abolition of quarantine in all British ports – including in Scotland. This came as a direct result of the 1892 epidemic which demonstrated what had already been known but had never been illuminated with such clarity, that having dual authority in the ports hindered the efficient working of both authorities. It also divided and muddied the integrity of the sanitary zone that had been constructed around the ports. During a crisis as potentially large as the 1892 epidemic, the cracks in the system were brought into sharp relief. As no threat on the scale of that posed in 1892 had arisen in the previous twenty years of the Port Sanitary Authorities' existence, the problems and rivalries between the two bodies could be accommodated for the appeasement of foreign pressures which demanded the continuation of quarantine and its structural operation (as discussed in the previous chapter). Yet, what was most politically fortuitous was that the 1892 epidemic clearly demonstrated that the quarantine employed in other countries to prevent the import of the disease had not proved successful. Thus, the ultimate proof of the superiority of the English System over quarantine appeared to have been confirmed, vindicating the British position at the International Sanitary Conferences over the previous four decades.

Some headway in international accord had begun to be reached just prior to the epidemic when another International Sanitary Conference had been held in Venice in January 1892. Again cholera was the focus of discussion, but this time with particular – almost exclusive – reference to the Suez Canal. For the first time an accord was composed which was signed by all the representative nations. Although the agreement somewhat compromised the British delegates' desire for completely free pratique in the Canal requiring some quarantine for suspected and infected vessels, it provided a welcome concession within the increasingly impossible impasse which had developed between British and French interests in the Canal. As *The Times* noted in February 1892, 'this is the first international sanitary conference which has adopted definite and complete regulations to improve the present state of things and safeguard the interests of trade conjointly with those of public health'.[73]

Not long after the 1892 epidemic, another International Conference was convened in Dresden in March 1893, and this time Britain was in a prime position, having been the least affected by the epidemic, to persuade the 'Quarantine States' to reconsider the English System. It meant that as far as Britain was concerned 'the conditions for the summoning of a Sanitary Conference were far more favourable than had been the case on former occasions'.[74] Furthermore, the 1892 conference, concerned more with Suez and having found an agreeable compromise on prophylaxis in the Canal, had set a precedent for consensus which had previously proved unattainable.

The final ratified convention, resulting from the 1893 conference in Dresden, saw further minor concessions to Britain's formerly uncompromising position, but it was generally regarded as having sufficiently incorporated the English System into international prophylaxis. Minimum and maximum periods for a 'quarantine of observation' were applied to healthy passengers from infected vessels, but because this 'observation' was not required to take place on board the vessel 'it will require no alteration whatever in the Cholera Regulations under which our ports are at present administered'.[75] Furthermore, only merchandise defined as 'susceptible' to 'contamination by choleraic matter', such as bed linen and clothing, was required to be detained or destroyed, and as such 'the convention offer[ed] advantages as regards the landing of merchandise which we trust will tend to free our commerce from some of the vexatious restrictions to which it has hitherto been so often subjected'.[76]

Despite these minor concessions, the British delegation refused to compromise on the issues of the new science of bacteriology. Eight years had passed since the notorious 1885 conference at which it was made clear that Britain would not entertain the practical – or political – implications of bacteriology for port health. These methods were becoming much more widespread by 1893, but British public health officials remained resolute. The 1892 epidemic had further demonstrated to British physicians involved in port disease control that the principles and practice of bacteriology could not prevent the import or spread of the disease. In Hamburg, for example, where bacteriological testing was employed from almost the first cases, more than 8,500 people died of the disease within the first month.[77] In English ports, on the other hand, the reliance on clinical diagnosis and on sanitary measures had effectively prevented the disease. Thorne Thorne, again sent to represent British interests at Dresden (but by this time also in his role as Chief Medical Officer of the Local Government Board), wrote to the Foreign Office in February 1893 to clarify the position which would be adopted by Britain at the conference:

> The verification by bacteriological examination and on the spot, of the precise nature of first 'choleraic' attacks is a requirement which Her Majesty's Government may hesitate to accept as a definite 'obligation'. Apart from possible questions as to its value from a scientific point of view, the interval of time involved in making the necessary investigation is more than likely to become associated with a delay in the adoption of the necessary measures of prevention, such as may be of serious import. For the purposes of notification and of prevention every case of choleraic diarrhoea should be regarded as one of cholera, and be forthwith dealt with as such.[78]

This not only allowed the fundamental concern of avoiding any delays to maritime trade to be protected but also maintained the assertion of a particular 'English' response to 'exotic' disease. The adoption and use or not of bacteriology had become an expression of sovereignty and political economy at the conferences. The way it coalesced with the management of the ports was a matter of great delicacy, where a rhetoric of its redundancy remained crucial while the politics of quarantine endured.

In the end, the convention which was successfully negotiated permitted some limited detention but finally appeared to vindicate the English System. Ships, having sailed from a cholera-infected port but not having on board any cases of the disease, i.e. 'suspected' vessels, were to be granted free pratique. They could, however, be detained at the discretion of the local authorities, but for no longer than a period of five days from the date of sailing. The passengers and crew of a vessel which had a case of cholera on board within the previous seven days, i.e. an 'infected' vessel, could be detained for a period of up to five days after the date of arrival. It was, however, included within the ratified agreement that 'no persons arriving in Great Britain in cholera-infected vessels, other than those who are actually sick on arrival, will be compulsorily detained'.[79] The detention, for purposes of medical observation, of any crew and passengers of 'infected' vessels was to occur, 'if possible', after disembarkation.

Not only did the convention appear to sanction the English System's removal of custodial medical observation and surveillance-based sanitary precautions, but it was also interpreted as an affirmation and triumph for its superiority and modernity:

> It appears that the application of the Convention will, in the more backward countries, meet with opposition from populations that have hitherto trusted to Quarantine Regulations, in the old sense of the term, to preserve them from cholera. In such countries the adoption of the Convention by Her Majesty's Government would, no doubt, be of value in strengthening the hands of those who are in favour of the sanitary system so long followed with success in this country, and it would afford to those countries a knowledge of security that their trade will, in the United Kingdom, continue to enjoy that freedom from useless restrictions which is guaranteed by the Convention.[80]

As *The Times* reported, the Dresden convention had finally achieved the general aims that Britain had advocated 'alone' since the first conference in 1851, and persuaded other European States to substitute 'the haphazard and arbitrary action of individual States and local authorities' for 'measures compatible with the necessities of international intercourse and commerce'.[81] The sanitary zone had been extended and sanctioned.

There was, however, one limitation to this, and one exception to the free pratique of healthy passengers arriving on non-infected vessels – migrants. Before departing for the conference, Thorne Thorne wrote to the President of the Local Government Board to say that, while he and his colleagues would object at all levels to quarantines and detentions which would disrupt the free movement of maritime traffic, he felt that it might, on the other hand, 'be undesirable to interpose objection to restriction of some sort being imposed ... as regards special classes of traffic'. He clarified his meaning of 'special classes of traffic' as 'restrictions ... aimed at preventing the undesirable immigration of destitute aliens from cholera stricken districts'.[82] Indeed, the conference agreed that local authorities would be granted the power to enact special regulations in the case of vessels which carried migrants and which, they qualified, were overcrowded and unsanitary.[83] This conflated 'infected' ports and ships, which were 'cholera stricken', with migrants and implied that they were, themselves, the location of disease. The undesirability of cholera was being disassociated from its 'foreign' origins and placed within the moving body of the migrant.

Increased powers to detain this 'special class of traffic' would permit Medical Officers working within the English System to regulate their movement within the sanitary zone; but this did not equate to quarantine. It did not come within the administration of the Quarantine Act, nor did it contradict Britain's other tradition of providing asylum. It was merely, as the *British Medical Journal* reported in August 1893, 'but a first line of defence' against 'the importation of pauper aliens, who [are] usually of the lowest class, coming from the most unsanitary districts'.[84] The detention of steerage-class migrants for observation at the ports, rather than releasing them into the responsibility of the local sanitary authorities, was, as the article continued, necessary for the following reasons:

> [they] are exceedingly likely to bring germs of disease, which, on account of the short passage, might not develop until they had left the ship, and they themselves had been lost sight of, in the poorest and most crowded portions of London. Since the present system has been in working order, this dangerous class has practically ceased to enter the port.[85]

Conclusion

The cholera epidemic of 1892 thus brought to the fore, for the first time, the particular issue of restricting entry to the United Kingdom to those immigrants whose standard of health was seen to be detrimental to the public health. Indeed, as the Cholera Prevention conference in late December 1892 determined, the strict enforcement of the Cholera Regulations was intended to deter the arrival of immigrants, where no other authority under the law was able. As Collingridge explained to his colleagues, 'This inspection is necessary not only for the detection of infected persons but also to prevent the importation of pauper aliens with the danger attendant thereon'.[86] And, for the moment, they appeared to succeed. Describing unequivocally the effect of the 1892 Cholera Order at the Cholera Prevention conference, Collingridge spoke approvingly of its consequence for migrants:

> COLLINGRIDGE: [The] arrangement had had the desired result, and one effect had been to check Jewish pauper immigration ... When the form[87] was filled up it was sent to the Sanitary Authority of the district in which the person said he resided, and that Authority was informed that he was detained on board the ship pending verification of the address. The passengers were kept on board the

ship practically as prisoners until an answer received from the Sanitary Authority by post or by wire.

DR. ARMSTRONG (PMOH Newcastle-on-Tyne): That system will soon stop the immigration of Jewish paupers.[88]

Indeed, these 'arrangements' were characterised in the United States as constituting a policy of immigration restriction. As the *New York Medical Journal* reported in September 1892, the insistence on verifiable addresses of immigrants as they arrived in the port was 'virtually a prohibition of immigration, as the question can hardly be answered by the average immigrant unless he is very carefully coached'.[89] As the example of the *Gemma* demonstrated, whether satisfactory or unsatisfactory, migrants' addresses were inconsequential to the decision made to detain them.

The 1892 epidemic thus not only brought changes – or at least provided a definite impetus to change – to the operation of port prophylaxis, it also began in Britain a new attitude to the restriction of immigration on medical grounds. It marked a pivotal moment in the orientation of public health concerns at the ports and the way they were regulated. These restrictions sat uncomfortably between a commitment to free pratique, a tradition of asylum and the desire to restrict the entry of undesirable and potentially 'disease-carrying' migrants. Although Britain remained committed after 1892 to maintaining the fluidity of the sanitary zone, allowing for the free movement of trading vessels, unhindered by the costly delays of maritime quarantines, the detention of vessels carrying third- or steerage-class migrants required a redefinition of that space. While being of little consequence epidemiologically in the British Isles, the 1892 epidemic had greatly significant implications for the plasticity and elasticity of the sanitary zone, reorienting the 'exoticness' of cholera away from 'foreign' ports and into the 'foreign' bodies of migrants. This not only helped to redistribute medical regulating authority at the ports away from the Customs Service and into the hands of the Port Sanitary Authorities, but it also began to change the direction of port disease control away from categories of 'place' ('infected' ports and vessels) toward categories of people (migrants, and racially and economically defined 'undesirables'). As the century drew to a close, neatly focused immigration control, rather than potentially open-ended quarantine, was starting to change the way lines of sovereignty were defined, while continuing to permit sufficient fluidity for the progress of non-migrant vessels.

Notes

1 R. Thorne Thorne, *Twenty-Second Annual Report of the LGB, 1892–3* – Supplement Containing the Report of the Medical Officer (London: HMSO, 1894) [C. 7412.], p. xxv.

2 A third origin, responsible for the East African epidemic, was identified as the 'Arabian' epidemic of 1890–91, which followed pilgrim routes to the 'Somali coast' of Africa, in the early summer of 1892. It was reported to have been re-imported, later in the year, back to Arabia. Thorne Thorne, *Annual Report LGB 1892–3*, p. xvii.

3 F.W. Barry, 'Report on the Origin and Progress of the Western Diffusion of Cholera During the Year 1892', *Annual Report of the LGB, 1892–3*, Appendix A. No. 12, p. 117.

4 Thorne Thorne, *Annual Report LGB 1892–3*, p. xvii.

5 The Pale of Settlement was created by imperial decree, and was that part of the Russian Empire within which Russia's Jewish population was required to live and work between the late eighteenth and early twentieth century.

6 Other immigrant groups settled in Britain at this time. Irish immigration, although not near to the scale of the 1840s and 1850s, was still ongoing. German clerical workers constituted a large proportion of immigrant numbers up until the late 1880s. Italians also immigrated, and Lithuanians were a proportionately significant immigrant group into Scotland. These immigrant groups, and others, continued to enter Britain from the early 1880s but, by the 1890s, were mostly eclipsed by the number of East European Jewish immigrants. Other European migrants often shared with the Jewish migrants the steerage accommodation of the migrant steamships.
   Holmes, *John Bull's Island*, pp. 20–31.

7 Leonard Shapiro, 'The Russian Background of the Anglo-American Jewish Immigration', in Colin Holmes (ed.), *Migration in European History*, vol. 1 (Cheltenham: Elgar Reference Collection, 1996).

8 Markel, *Quarantine!*, p. 141.

9 *Ibid.*, p. 86.

10 *Ibid.*

11 Evans, *Death in Hamburg*, p. 230.

12 *Ibid.*, p. 286.

13 *Ibid.*, p. 292.

14 *Ibid.*, p. 316.

15 Belvidere, opened in 1870, was Glasgow's central municipal fever (infectious disease) hospital.

16 *Glasgow Medical Journal*, 38, 3 (Sept. 1892), p. 208.

17 Thorne Thorne, *Annual Report LGB 1892–3*, p. xxiii.

18 *BMJ*, 10 Sept. 1892, p. 604.

19 *Ibid.*

20 *BMJ*, 17 Sept. 1892, p. 658.

21 Markel, *Quarantine!*, p. 87.

22 Paul Weindling, 'A Virulent Strain: German Bacteriology as Scientific Racism, 1890–1920', in Ernst and Harris (eds), *Race, Science and Medicine, 1700–1960*, 218–34, p. 226.

23 Paul Weindling, *Epidemics and Genocide in Eastern Europe, 1890–1945* (Oxford: Oxford University Press, 2000), p. 62.

24 *Ibid.*, p. 63.

25 *Ibid.*

26 *Ibid.*

27 Letter from Lord Salisbury to Thorne Thorne and E.H. Philips, 17 May 1892, NA, FO146/3346.

28 See Hardy, 'Cholera', pp. 263–8.

29 Milne, 'Institutions,' p. 266

30 *The Lancet*, 10 Sept. 1892, p. 614.

31 *The Lancet*, 3 Sept. 1892, p. 592 (my italics).

32 *BMJ*, 10 Sept. 1892, p. 608.

33 *The Lancet*, 10 Sept. 1892, p. 614.

34 *The Times*, 1 Sept. 1892, p. 4a.

35 *Cholera Precautions for 1893 – Conference of Port Medical Officers of Health*, Reprinted from the 'Shipping and Mercantile Gazette', 17th December 1892, By Order of the Port of London Sanitary Committee, p. 6, CLRO, MISC MSS/337/3.

36 Quarantine Act, 1825 (6 Geo. III c.78), XVII.

37 *Cholera Precautions for 1893*, p. 76, CLRO, MISC MSS/337/3.

38 This applied to all classes of passengers arriving from foreign ports. However, the addresses of first and second class passengers were not questioned.

39 *Cholera Regulations*, Local Government Board, Whitehall, 29 Aug. 1892, NA, MH19/244.

40 'Monthly Report of the Port Medical Officer of Health', Oct., 1892, CLRO, *PSCP* (Oct. – Dec., 1892).

41 *Ibid.*

42 'Complaints of the German YMCA, London', letter dated, 24 Apr. 1893, CLRO, *PSCP* (June–Aug., 1893).

43 Letter dated, 27 Apr. 1893, *Ibid.*

44 Letter dated, 17 May 1893, *Ibid.*

45 No further information about this witness is provided beyond the testimony given here.

46 'Monthly Report of the Port Medical Officer of Health', Oct., 1892, CLRO, *PSCP* (Oct.–Dec., 1892).

47 *BMJ*, 10 Sept. 1892, p. 607.

48 NA MH55/897.

49 Barry, 'Report on the Origin and Progress', p. 182.

50 *Ibid.*

51 Telegram from Klein to LGB, 8 Aug. 1894, NA MH19/236.

52 *The Lancet*, 3 Sept. 1892, p. 593 (my italics).

53 'Medical Report from Hospital, Gravesend', CLRO, *PSCP* (July–Sept., 1892), 6 Sept. 1892.

54 *The Lancet*, 1 Oct. 1892, p. 783 (my italics).

55 See for example, 'Appendium Report on *Gemma*', CLRO, *PSCP* (July–Sept., 1892), Aug. 1892.

56 See for example, Telegram, 25 Aug. 1892, NA MH55/897.

57 Telegram, 26 Aug. 1892, NA MH55/897.

58 *The Times*, 9 Sept. 1892, p. 4b.

59 *N.Y. Med. Jnl.*, 1 Oct 1892, vol. 56, p. 385.

60 *Cholera Precautions for 1893*, CLRO, MISC MSS/337/1.

61 *Ibid.*

62 *Cholera Precautions for 1893*, pp. 2–3, CLRO, MISC MSS/337/3.

63 *Ibid.*, pp. 66–7.

64 *Ibid.*, pp. 4–5.

65 *Ibid.*, p. 49.

66 *Ibid.*, p. 69.

67 *Ibid.*, p. 6.

68 *Ibid.*, p. 8.

69 3 Oct. 1893, SRA CE60/1/89 p. 197.

70 *Ibid.*

71 In September 1893 the ports listed as 'infected' by the Glasgow and Greenock Sanitary Authorities were: Antwerp, Palermo, Nantes, Rotterdam, Hamburg, Leghorn, Brest, Bilbao [various ports in] Algeria, St. Petersburg, and San Sebastian. *Ibid.*, p 194.

72 *Ibid.*, p. 201.

73 *The Times*, 1 Feb. 1892, p. 5e.

74 *Correspondence Respecting the Sanitary Convention, Signed at Dresden on April 15, 1893* (London: HMSO, 1893) [C. 7156], p. 37.

75 'Report of the British Delegates to the International Sanitary Conference of Dresden', *Twenty-Third Annual Report of the LGB, 1893–94 – Supplement Containing the Report of the Medical Officer* (London: HMSO, 1894) [C. 7538], Appendix A, No. 20, p. 455.

76 *Ibid.*, p. 456.

77 Evans, *Death in Hamburg*, p. 295, Table 4.

78 Letter from Thorne Thorne to Foreign Office, 13 Feb. 1893, NA MH19/238/14844/93.

79 *Ibid.*, p. 38.

80 Letter from 'Foreign Office to Local Government Board' – as well as Board of Trade and Admiralty – dated 11 May 1893, *Ibid.*, p. 37.

81 *The Times*, April 20, 1893 p. 5d.

82 Letter from Thorne Thorne to the President of the Local Government Board, dated 1 Jan. 1893, NA MH 19/238/664/93.

83 'British Delegates to the Dresden Sanitary Conference to the Earl of Rosebery', dated 18 April 1893, *Correspondence Respecting the Sanitary Convention*, p. 10.

84 *BMJ*, 5 Aug. 1893, p. 343.

85 *Ibid.*

86 Letter from Collingridge to Port Sanitary Committee, CLRO, *PSCP* (January–March 1893), 3 Jan. 1893.

87 Recording the intended accommodations of the migrants.

88 *Cholera Precautions for 1893*, pp. 12–13, CLRO, MISC MSS/337/3 (PMOH = Port Medical Officer of Health).

89 *New York Medical Journal*, 3 Sept. 1892, vol. 56. p. 251.

4

American ports in the sanitary zone

The cholera epidemic of 1892 brought the perceived threat of immigrant disease squarely within the purview of the sanitary system. Yet, over the following decade another factor influenced the increasing role of migrants in the development of port health and its intersection with immigration control. Just as the practice and policies of quarantine and the English System had responded to both internal and external stimuli, the formulation of a rhetoric of risk about migrants was similarly generated.

Greater than any other external source, American management of disease control and immigration restriction (particularly after 1891) influenced Britain's changing approach to port health and the 'alien problem'.[1] Maritime disease control and immigration restriction were closely linked in the United States. Systems of disease prevention were central tools in the defining of the national boundary, screening arrivals for so-called 'undesirables', and defining who could and who could not gain entrance to the country. These had direct repercussions in Britain. Of the 2.4 million Russian and Polish migrants who immigrated to the United States between 1881 and 1914,[2] approximately one million transmigrated through Britain.[3] However, the stricter immigration laws of the United States often encouraged migrants who fell short of the entry requirements to stay in Britain, either temporarily or on a permanent basis. More significantly, anxiety had grown in Britain over the conviction that a number of migrants who were rejected by US immigration officials were ending up in cities like London or Liverpool.

The United States also influenced the way that Britain dealt with the perceived health problems posed by immigrants by way of example. As the United States received by far the greatest number of migrants, pressure to create legislation for monitoring or restricting their arrival was exerted earlier in America than it was in Britain. Thus American legislation served, as John Garrard has suggested, as 'a blue-print for anti-alien agitators in England'.[4]

Similarly, as the progress and consequence of American policy and practice were observed in Britain, the conditions of British ports were also closely monitored in America. Applying what Aristede Zolberg has called 'remote control',[5] the United States established systems of inspection – and compelled shipping companies to do the same – at ports and frontiers of departure. This resulted in a heightened awareness of immigrant health screening at foreign ports and highlighted Britain's contrasting lack of similar control mechanisms at places of entry.

For these reasons, British public health and port authorities, as well as an increasing chorus of anti-alienists, directed their gaze across the Atlantic, seeking to define not only the solution to migrant-borne disease, but also the nature of the problem itself. This was reflected back across the ocean as the United States attempted to control the west-ward traffic of potential immigrants leaving their final ports of depar-ture. The space Britain negotiated at the littoral consequently required not only the largely eastward looking trade imperatives which had shaped its responses to quarantine and sanitation for most of the cen-tury, it also needed to accommodate an increasingly demanding trans-Atlantic response to European migration.

Defining American medical borders

The development of American policies and attitudes toward immigra-tion since the late nineteenth century has long attracted the work of historians. Much of it has focused on the creation of an American 'identity' and the formulation of both land and sea borders, examining different mechanisms of regulation from labour control to medical restriction. More recently, scholars have begun to look at the intercon-nectedness of US immigration with the policies of different states and private enterprise, and the global nature of migration.[6] Through the extension of systems of inspection to ports and frontiers in other parts of the globe, nineteenth- and early-twentieth-century American immi-gration regulation was not a process confined simply at the nation's geographical borders. These regulations relied upon distant US Consuls and, increasingly, privately owned shipping companies to carry out a 'remote border control', rejecting immigrants even before they boarded trans-continental railways or trans-Atlantic ships. Zolberg traces this practice back to the immigration laws of the early to mid-nineteenth century.[7]

While these were mostly legislated at the state level, controlling aspects of immigrant arrival and passage, the American demand for labour through most of the century encouraged the continuation of relatively open door policies.[8] Only later in the century did the federal government pass legislation which restricted entry to the country, starting in 1882 with the Chinese Exclusion Act as well as the Immigration Act of that year. The latter refused entry to immigrants thought to be convicted felons, 'lunatics', paupers, or otherwise at risk of becoming a public charge and levied a fifty cent duty on every incoming migrant. Although legislated at the federal level, inspections were carried out by individual states, and in order to avoid possible deportation from ports of arrival in America, were increasingly carried out by transportation companies operating in Europe. In 1891 the regulation of immigration was finally brought within the sole remit of the federal government with the Immigration Act, 1891. Amy Fairchild has effectively argued that the Act was essentially intended to control the labour market, utilising its various categories of 'desirability' and 'undesirability' as mechanisms of inclusion as much as exclusion.[9] One of the central categories defined by the Act was 'persons suffering from a loathsome or dangerous contagious disease'. Fairchild explains that, 'In the specific context of immigration control, the metaphors of disease and immigration not only expressed nativist fears of contamination but also and more critically the need to order and manage ...'[10] This ordering and management was about identifying those who were not fit for inclusion as well as serving as a 'normative exercise'[11] for those who were. Those rejected by Public Health Service inspectors were required to be returned to their port of origin by the steamship company which carried them to America. It was these restrictions that to a large extent put American 'remote control' into practice, setting in place a system whereby 'migrants were rejected at the German–Russian and German–Austrian borders, or prevented from boarding trans-Atlantic steamships at European ports because the American immigration inspectors *might* refuse to admit them'.[12]

In addition to immigration controls, American ports were guarded against the possible importation of disease by traditional quarantines. Quarantine was enforced under the Quarantine Act of 1878 until the passing of the National Quarantine Act in early 1893. The 1878 Act was the first attempt at applying a national approach to quarantine and had been established in response to an epidemic of yellow fever.[13] Any immigrant or vessel infected with a contagious disease, or proceeding from an infected port, was prevented under the Act from entering any US port without first undergoing a medical inspection and a period of quarantine where required. Although it was a federal act it could not ordinarily supersede or interfere with sanitary procedures or quarantine systems already in operation in individual states or municipal authorities. Thus, the implementation of any quarantine measures ultimately remained under the regulation of state or municipal authorities.[14] Nevertheless, the 1878 Act permitted the federal government to enforce additional quarantine regulations at individual ports in the event of an emergency. These powers were further enforced with the passing of the National Board of Health Act, 1879, which, although providing little other real authority to the Board of Health, permitted this federal agency to take over the quarantine responsibilities of any state if their own laws proved ineffectual.[15]

The National Board of Health Act was primarily concerned with preventing 'the introduction of infectious and contagious diseases', with specific reference to the 'extensive prevalence of yellow fever in certain parts of this ... and the almost continual existence of the danger of the introduction of such contagious or infectious diseases as yellow fever and cholera by vessels coming to this country from infected ports abroad.'[16] The Act required that all ships departing from a foreign port bound for America were required to be in possession of a Bill of Health and 'sanitary history' endorsed by a US Consular Official or Medical Officer working in the country of departure.[17] This required the Consular Official to inspect the ship and port of departure, as well as any Bill of Health or inspection which had been made by a port official belonging to the country of departure. It was believed that this would render Bills of Health more reliable as the authorities of the country of departure might possibly conceal epidemic infections in order to protect their own commercial interests.[18]

As discussed in chapter 2, in order to implement this essential feature of the National Board of Health Act, the United States required international sanction – to which end the 1881 Washington International Sanitary Conference was called. For the Americans, the conference sought to reach an agreement which would ensure a level of cleanliness and sanitation on board vessels before departure. US delegates framed their argument in terms of preventing obstructions to commerce through the time-consuming and costly enforcement of quarantine in America which would necessarily be applied to ships whose health status was questionable. The success of their argument was, however, limited. The British delegates were among the chief opponents to the American proposal, labelling it impracticable. Again, as at the 1866 and 1874 conferences, the British argued that the suggestion of an 'independent' medical inspection of vessels greatly undermined and questioned the authority of British Medical Officers, and they refused to support the proposal. In the end no effective resolutions or international agreements were reached, except that US consuls were permitted to endorse Bills of Health prepared by health officials of the country of departure. Although this was not the ideal outcome from the American point of view, it did allow the United States to oversee foreign departures and maintain most of the clauses under the National Board of Health Act and the 1878 Quarantine Act.

So, 'remote control' was a function of both immigration and quarantine laws, ensuring that the regulation of healthy and unhealthy bodies wishing to enter America was a far-reaching enterprise. American medical borders therefore extended well beyond the geographical borders of the United States and defined a space where categories of 'desirability' and 'undesirability' determined progress into and through that space. It reached across and to the frontiers of American and foreign states and created overlapping and sometimes conflicting bounds of sovereignty.

American medical borders and 'England'

The transcursion of American border controls into and through 'English' territory had a significant effect on attitudes to immigration and health in British ports. Alison Bashford has convincingly argued that settler colonies such as Australia, New Zealand and the Cape Colony were influential in the development of changing British attitudes towards immigration.[19] However, the perceived and real practical implications of American 'remote control' meant that the United States exerted the greatest influence on Britain in relation to the regulation of immigration in this period. One of the most notable ramifications of American law for Britain was the authority both state and federal laws had for returning migrants deemed 'undesirable' to their last port of departure. 'Undesirability' was measured both by economic and medical factors although neither was grounds for rejection under British law. When immigrants were rejected, either on arrival in the United States or for offences committed within a year of arrival, the steamship company which had brought them to America was responsible for returning them to their port or frontier of origin. Frequently, in order to avoid the full cost of the passage back to Eastern and Central Europe, companies economised by returning the migrants to their last port of departure at less distant British ports. This point was noted some years later in the evidence of a Medical Officer and Ophthalmic surgeon to the Royal Commission on Alien Immigration in 1903:

> ...cases had been referred to me which had been returned from America, aliens who had gone to America, and had been examined by the immigration officers at certain ports in America, and sent back, not to Poland, but to London. So that there is a possibility of them accumulating in this country, on account of the fact that the shipping companies find it cheaper to send them back to London than to Poland.[20]

The passage back to Britain was not only cheaper but also, as an investigation undertaken by the Poor Jews Temporary Shelter in London discovered, better for business:

> If they went back to their own countries rejected by the United States it would considerably affect [the shipping agent's] business in those countries; and as a result they come to England and learning from the agents here that they can get to America through Canada they either take this course or remain in London.[21]

Attempting to avoid the expensive liability they incurred, shipping company owners undertook to enforce medical inspections of their own before departure and refused to carry migrants who would not, on arrival in the United States, pass the increasingly rigorous requirements of entry:

> While at the boarding-house [in Liverpool], the immigrant is under constant medical surveillance; for the shipping companies employ a medical man (some companies employing a special 'shore doctor' others sending the surgeon of the ship in which the immigrants are to sail), whose duty it is to pay a daily visit to the boarding-houses and to inquire into the health of their inmates. One principal object

of this medical inspection is to avoid all risk of shipping persons whose state of health might cause danger or inconvenience to their fellow passengers. But the inspection serves at the same time to enable the discovery of persons who are likely to be treated as ineligible by the American immigration authorities by reason of their state of health[22]

This and the return to British ports of migrants who had been deemed not fit to settle in the United States was perceived by many as not only posing a financial burden but also as threatening the public health. Yet, despite the great concern raised by this issue, as expressed in the media and particularly by those opposed to unrestricted immigration, the numerical impact of returned and remaining migrants was minimal. In 1893 the Board of Trade appointed two men, John Burnett and David Schloss, to compile a report on the legal, economic and social aspects of immigration in the United States.[23] The report was commissioned both on the impetus of parliamentary discussion on the issue of alien immigration into Britain, and because the duty bestowed on the Board of Trade to compile statistics relating to immigration had, during the course of numerous inquiries, left the Board of Trade with 'a great deal' of information about immigration to the United States. Although the majority of the report was concerned with the internal workings of American immigration policy, Schloss included a subsection titled *Effect of United States Laws Upon Ratepayers in United Kingdom*.[24] This examined the extent to which persons debarred or expelled from the United States within a year of settlement, and who were 'returned' to Britain, subsequently sought public relief.

Schloss reported that a total of 118 immigrants from New York, Boston and Philadelphia, both rejected on arrival and returned during the year 1892,[25] were conveyed to ports in Britain at the expense of the steamship companies.[26] Of the eighty-five returned from New York, sixty-five had migrated from Russia or Poland, twelve from Germany, six from Sweden and the rest from other Northern European countries such as Finland. As Table 4.1 clearly illustrates, both the actual number returned to British ports and the percentage this represented of the total arrivals into the three American ports was very low.

The eighty-five immigrants returned to Britain from New York during 1892 represented only three per cent of the 2,574 who were

Table 4.1 Returns to UK ports[27]

1892	New York	Boston	Philadelphia	Total: NY, Boston, Philadelphia
Total no. of alien steerage arrivals	374,741	29,709	29,292	433,742
No. returned to UK ports from the United States	85	27	6	118
Percentage of total arrivals returned to UK ports	0.02	0.09	0.02	0.03

debarred or returned within a year of arriving in New York.[28] The 2,489 who were not returned to Britain were taken back to European departure ports. A similar proportion was returned to the Continent from Boston and Philadelphia. Furthermore, as Schloss noted, 'a very considerable proportion' of the migrants who were returned to British ports was subsequently returned to their respective continental ports of origin.[29] According to Board of Trade reports for England (not including London) only three returned immigrants, all in Liverpool, became reliant on public relief in institutions maintained by the local rates. In Scotland, although total numbers are not given, four returned immigrants sought public assistance in 1892, all within the Parish of Govan Combination.[30]

Application to poor relief funds by returned migrants was infrequent, and once a claim was made the expense was often reimbursed by either the shipping company or, in the case of Jewish migrants, by local Jewish charitable organisations. Yet, regardless of their infrequency, as described by Schloss and demonstrated through an examination of poor relief applications in Glasgow,[31] the belief that migrants, who were unwanted by America, were publicly supported by local ratepayers was a powerful one. Two examples demonstrate the type of relief afforded to this conspicuous few.

Goldie Friedman, a twenty-seven-year-old Russian Jewish woman, was brought before the Glasgow Parish of Govan Combination with an application for poor relief by State Line Company Officials on 23 February 1886:

this woman was an emigrant on her way to America and turned insane on board the vessel. She was three weeks confined in an asylum at Staten Island, America, and was handed back to the State Line Company, who now applies for her removal to asylum. She having arrived at Mavis Bank Quay on board the *S.S. State of Georgia*. Her husband is in Baltimore. Sent to Merryflats [asylum] and removed on 12th March by order of the board.[32]

She remained in the asylum for nearly three weeks, the cost of which was claimed from the State Line Company.[33] Similarly, the Allan Line Company met the cost of five days spent in the Poorhouse by Abraham Wahlhandler in October 1891. He had been in America for four months but had been 'Returned by authorities from New York'. His only ailment appears to have been a sprained ankle, yet he was 'refused at Royal Infirmary not requiring surgical treatment' and thus applied for [outdoor medical] poor relief.[34]

So, although American policy to return to shipping companies any immigrant expelled on grounds of health or likely to become a public charge attracted both popular and some official attention in Britain, the quantitative evidence is unable to account for the strength of the reaction. Rather, what lay behind it was the idea that the absence of immigration control in Britain allowed entry to people who had been rejected by the United States for failing to satisfy its requirements for permanent settlement – being physically, morally or economically 'undesirable'. These 'undesirables' were not only permitted to enter Britain, but also to settle, work and claim relief. An article in the *British Medical Journal* in 1896 complained that 'hundreds of thousands of wretched paupers ... are crowded together in the cities of the Pale until life becomes intolerable. Then they escape in hordes in the hope of reaching the free West. The stronger and more able-bodied manage to reach America, but the less fit stay behind in England'.[35]

This notion that Britain received those immigrants who US immigration officials rejected came to the fore in the British medical and popular press in 1892 and remained contentious over the following decade. Part of the concern, despite the preventive system established at British ports, was that no medical inspection was undertaken on vessels departing American ports for Britain and Europe. While inspections – established under the National Board of Health Act – were carried out on all vessels bound for the United States before embarkation, none were on those returning. As a

Medical Inspector working with the US Consul in Britain wrote to the Board of Trade in 1896,

> passengers leaving the other side are not required to undergo an examination at all, as the object of the American Government is simply to prevent disease being imported into their own country, and they apparently do not care what disease may break out in the ship or may be imported into this country.[36]

The US border, even as it extended to 'remote' frontiers, appeared all the more rigid and impermeable in 1892 when the new United States Immigration Act of 1891, combined with state quarantine laws, was put to the test with the arrival of cholera from Europe. This had particular consequences for Britain. While British officials anticipated the arrival of cholera, watching its progression across Europe 'from Whitehall' with limited alarm and urging local authorities 'to complete their sanitary defences in time to repel the threatened invasion',[37] America responded with considerably less restraint. As in Britain, the source of the disease was seen to be East European migrants, and the United States reacted with great vigour by initially focusing prevention almost exclusively on this group. As *The New York Times* noted, 'These people are offensive enough at best; under the present [cholera] circumstances, they are a positive menace to the health of the country'.[38]

The first cases of cholera arrived in New York on 30 August aboard the steamship *Moravia* sailing from Hamburg. The vessel was at once placed in quarantine with all passengers, regardless of health, detained upon it. With the arrival of more infected vessels imminent, President Harrison summoned a meeting with the Attorney General, Secretary of the Treasury and Supervising Surgeon General of the Marine Health Service. They agreed to impose from 1 September an extended period of quarantine – twenty days – on all vessels from infected ports which carried 'Russian Hebrew' immigrants. The period of quarantine applied only to immigrant steerage passengers; other passengers of cabin class would be released. The 1878 Quarantine Act permitted the federal government to impose periods of quarantines on vessels arriving in American ports during emergencies. Using this authority Harrison issued a circular which placed all responsibility for the importation of cholera on steerage class immigrants and the vessels which carried them. The circular referred specifically to the 'prevalence' of cholera in 'Russia, Germany and France, and at certain ports in Great Britain' and that 'immigrants in large numbers are coming into the United States from the infected districts aforesaid'.[39] It ordered, 'that no vessel from any foreign port carrying emigrants shall be permitted to enter any port of the United States until the said vessel has undergone quarantine detention for a period of twenty days'.[40]

As Howard Markel points out, this quarantine and the circular which enforced it 'had nothing to do with bacteriological concepts of cholera culture diagnosis or incubation periods. It was explicitly conceived as a financial brake to halt steerage immigration'.[41] With developments in bacteriological understanding of cholera in the United States, the estimated time deemed appropriate for the isolation of people who had been in contact with the disease was five to eight days.[42] Indeed, at the beginning of September 1892 the Advisory Medical Council of the Chamber of Commerce in New York[43] recommended that 'the period of quarantine detention of healthy persons ... should be five days in case no cholera occurs among them'.[44] However, President Harrison made it clear in his final two addresses to Congress that he strongly supported restrictions to the immigration of Russian Jews. The twenty-day quarantine period on all steerage passengers and the vessels they arrived in was imposed, as Markel explains, not simply to provide New York with the greatest level of protection against cholera, but to drastically limit the number of immigrants who arrived. By enforcing such extended delays it would not be economically viable for steamship companies to continue to run the trans-Atlantic migrant routes. The scheme worked. Steamship companies which had first- and second-class bookings began to refuse to take on board steerage class immigrants and were subsequently spared the imposition and expense of quarantine.[45] In an attempt to re-establish steerage passage the steamship companies proposed to the US Consul in Liverpool an expansion of the steam disinfection facilities for cleansing steerage-class clothing and baggage in order to eliminate cholera. But this

> experiment proved that to continue the steaming properly would necessitate great enlargement of the plant at considerable expense, and as it was believed that even with this precaution the twenty days' quarantine at United States ports would still be required, the steamship companies concluded to abandon it.[46]

After the failure of this proposal all steerage passengers already booked aboard vessels sailing from Liverpool to America were removed from ships carrying first- and second-class passengers and, 'the emigrants thus shut out with others whom the companies had already contracted to carry are being sent over in special ships with no other passengers.'[47] The Consul at Liverpool then issued orders to all steamship companies operating out of the port not to book steerage emigrants until further notification and to 'avoid taking first and second class passengers from infected ports.'[48]

If the cessation of European immigration was Harrison's intention in imposing such a severe and focused quarantine policy, his scheme proved successful. Russian Jewish immigrants arriving in New York averaged approximately 3,800 per month during the early months of 1892, but between October and December, after the application of immigrant quarantine, this average fell to around 270 a month.[49] The policy was not entirely successful in preventing the spread of the disease into the city of New York but unlike previous epidemics, such as the epidemic of 1849 which killed 5,017 New Yorkers within three months,[50] there were only nine deaths from cholera reported beyond the infected ships in the City of New York during September 1892.[51]

The decline in the number of migrant passengers arriving in New York in September 1892 corresponded with and contributed to a decline in the number of migrants who arrived in Britain. Medical officers working at British ports and for the Local Government Board – Thorne Thorne and Collingridge for example – saw the decline in numbers arriving into British ports in 1892 as a reflection of the Local Government Board's Cholera Orders of that summer.[52] However, the rigid restrictions of American 'remote control' at European ports and Continental frontiers,[53] particularly during the cholera epidemic, were probably more responsible for the decline. The *British Medical Journal* remarked,

> if evidence were needed of the effect produced by the drastic measures of quarantine adopted by America during the prevailing cholera epidemic upon the flow of Russo-Jewish transmigrants from Hamburg across Great Britain on their way to the West, it may be found in the return of the Board of Trade as to the number of aliens arriving at ports in the United Kingdom during the past month. In place of the 5,615 aliens who landed on our shores from Hamburg *en route* for America in September of 1891, there was not one such entry in the same month of the present year.[54]

The inspection and confinement of migrants in Hamburg and other parts of Continental Europe during the outbreak combined with Harrison's twenty-day quarantine to greatly reduce trans-Atlantic migration that year. However, even though migrant numbers in British,

US and European ports were drastically cut, and cities like New York were relatively untouched by the epidemic, in Britain quarantine still represented the 'evils' long associated with it: its essential ineffectiveness and its ability to incite panic.

The treatment of one particular vessel in New York during the epidemic came to symbolise the characterisation of quarantine as excessive and unreasonable that had become standard rhetoric in Britain. The New York epidemic did not extend much beyond the end of September, but during that month seven ships heavily infected with cholera arrived in New York Harbour. Their combined mortality reached 120 people and their remaining passengers and crew were detained in quarantine, along with thousands more from other vessels that arrived into the port. On 5 September, two ships, the *Rugia* and the *Normannia*, arrived at the harbour from Hamburg with cholera on board. On the same day, more passengers aboard the *Moravia* succumbed to the disease. Desperately over-stretched, the Health Officer of the Port of New York, William T. Jenkins, decided to place the entire population of the *Normannia*, 1,355 people, in quarantine.[55] However, the port's quarantine facilities at Hoffman and Swinburne islands were already dreadfully overcrowded with cholera victims and suspects and the port itself was getting more congested with arriving vessels requiring inspection and detention. Not willing to wait until the federal government could provide additional space, Jenkins coordinated the purchase and preparation of a hotel for quarantine accommodation on Fire Island, thirty miles east of New York City.[56] However, on arrival at Fire Island the passengers of the *Normannia* were forced to remain on the pleasure boat which had ferried them from New York. For three days a combination of bad weather and irate local residents on Long Island prohibited their landing at the temporary quarantine barracks and forced them to remain on board without even the most basic amenities.

The incident caused national and international outrage and the world's press seized upon the affair. In Britain, it was extensively covered in *The Times* and in medical journals such as *The Lancet* which was particularly critical of the quarantine policy and its consequences:

> If healthy people are, in the eyes of the [United States] Government, such a danger to a community because they come from an infected port, or because cholera has occurred on board the ships in which they travel, that they must be kept away for ten or twenty days, although this may involve the greatest cruelties, indecencies and danger of death, then why complain of the action of people such as

those who, in the Fire Island case, armed with clubs, pistols, boat-
hooks and rifles, and were deaf to the entreaties, tears and pleadings
of helpless women and children, who, though healthy, had been
labelled by the quarantine system as dangerous?[57]

The incident seemed to provide the ultimate, dramatic evidence
against quarantine. It had all the necessary ingredients to demonstrate
the claims its British opponents had been making throughout the century – insalubrious accommodations, an angry mob – and offered a
perfect counterpoint to the enlightened practice of the English System.
For those who still advocated the detention of vessels arriving from
cholera-infected ports, *The Lancet* presented the example of the
Normannia in warning:

> We would urge people who are thus pressing the [British] Govern-
> ment [to 'authorise a reversion to the ancient, useless, and cruel sys-
> tem known as "quarantine"'] to read again the intelligence from Fire
> Island, and also note that the practical outcome of the New York
> quarantine system is an announcement on authority of the Board of
> Health that five cases of genuine Asiatic Cholera have already
> occurred in New York.[58]

The incident and the surrounding events of 1892 prompted further discussion and review of immigration restriction and quarantine laws in
the United States, as it had in Britain. Yet, in contrast to Britain, rather
than discouraging the use of quarantine, the epidemic instigated a debate
in the United States which led to the passing of the 1893 Quarantine Act,
which extended the use of quarantine, making it a federal, rather than
state, responsibility. American medical borders thus became more
tightly defined and the health of those who could cross them was more
critically judged, helping, as Alexandra Minna Stern explained in reference to the Mexican border some decades later, 'to solidify a boundary
line that had previously been much more indistinct'.[59]

In general, British and American positions regarding the effectiveness and desirability of quarantine were at odds with one another. In
Britain, the application of quarantine was thought to be archaic and
ineffectual, while in the United States it was believed to be the safest
and most assured means of preventing the importation of infectious
disease. Neither position, however, was necessarily related to consensus or majority medical understanding. As Markel points out: 'it was
not Jenkins' (or any other health official's) scientific understanding of
cholera that would primarily guide the management of the epidemic.

Bacteriological knowledge had far less to do with the proceedings of the 1892 epidemics than politics and nativistic sentiments'[60] The definition of national boundaries through the regulation of borders closely tied quarantine to immigration. Any discussion about quarantine in 1890s America was not only a discussion about how to prevent the importation of disease, but also about how to prevent the importation of a certain class of immigrant, increasingly identified through logics of health and illness. As Markel argues,

> Vibrant and colorful in its expression, but often blurred at the edges, the medical profession's debate [about quarantine] had less to do with the victory of germ theory and the institution of the laboratory in public health than with the bitter fight over U.S. immigration policy.[61]

In its rigid designation of 'desirable' and 'undesirable' bodies and newly consolidated role as a framer of national space, the 1893 Quarantine Act was largely perceived as an attempt at both disease prevention and at immigration control. It achieved the latter, however, under the more palatable guise of public health.[62] Ironically, given the approach during the 1892 epidemic, it was based less on a policy of total isolation and non-intercourse than had existed under the separate state regulations. Instead, the Act appeared to adopt a system that looked more like the British System of 'medical inspection, rigid sanitary regulations, and the isolation of those found to be ill'[63] The differences in port prophylaxis, then, were perhaps more about rhetoric and posturing than practical solutions.

Even so, similar to European critics, many interested Americans commented on the particular importance of free trade doctrine in the differently developing system of disease control at British ports. The 'worship of the Mammon of pounds, shillings and pence,'[64] they remarked with scorn, sought the least expensive and most efficient method of intercepting infection. Trading interests rather than science, they argued, underlay the English System. In an article entitled 'The Ability of the State to Prevent an Epidemic of Cholera' which appeared in the Philadelphia journal, *Medical News* in September 1892, Benjamin Lee, the Secretary to the State Board of Health of Pennsylvania, offered, for example, a blunt reading of the British response to the threat of cholera:

> The system of seacoast quarantine in Great Britain, as has long been known to American sanitarians, is defective in the extreme. Recent

disclosures have developed the fact that there is really no power in the Government to enforce quarantine. The great British doctrine of free trade seems to have been pushed to its utmost limit to include disease as well as other commodities.[65]

However, Lee admitted that throughout the previous weeks, while the United States had struggled to keep down the number of cholera cases breaking through the barriers of quarantine, the British System had proved more successful in preventing the spread of the disease. Yet such a system, where 'everything [was] in such an admirable condition of cleanliness and [had] such strict enforcement of local precautions that the germs will quickly die', required 'a complete and thorough sanitary organisation of the country so that no foot of ground escapes frequent sanitary inspection and no accumulation of filth is allowed to remain on its surface or beneath the surface for an hour'. Within two paragraphs of having condemned the mercenary impetus of disease control at Britain's ports, Lee shifted his position to one of admiration as he lamented the deficiencies of the American system. 'Such, unfortunately, is not the sanitary organisation of the States of this Union'.[66]

British sanitation was admired, envied and sought to be emulated. Those in the United States who favoured sanitary control rather than quarantine looked not only to Britain but also its colonies. India, in particular, was used as an illustration of how simple sanitary precautions could drastically reduce the risk of infectious disease spreading in notoriously 'filthy' cities. Night-soil collection was a case in point. According to a contributor to the *North American Review*, this was the type of reform which was required – and certainly possible – in cities such as New York if sanitation was to be relied upon to prevent imported disease.[67]

However, for some the English System was in no way desirable. S.T. Armstrong, a visiting physician to the Harlem Hospital, wrote an article for the *New York Medical Journal* in September 1892 entitled 'Quarantine and the Present Status of Quarantine Laws'.[68] Armstrong asserted that in contrast with Britain 'the welfare of the many must be given precedence over the inconvenience of the few'.[69] He argued that the system which operated in Britain was in no way superior to the system of quarantine in place in the United States:

They profess to base their indifference to a quarantine in general to the improved sanitary conditions of their cities, towns and villages. And yet it is difficult to understand a sentiment that professes to

ignore a maritime quarantine, and yet provides a maritime inspection service, with crude appliances for caring for the sick who are
detained from an infected vessel.[70]

Arguing that the English System was little more than a second-rate
alternative to quarantine, Armstrong's central argument stressed that
quarantine was still used and indeed favoured as a preventative meas-
ure in Britain where there were no consequences for trade. He cited
the example of the quarantining of school children who had been
exposed to infectious disease and asked how British politicians and
public health authorities could support this when they frowned upon
maritime quarantine:

> The code of rules of the English Medical Officers of Schools Asso-
> ciation provides that a quarantine of from twelve to twenty-one
> days, according to the disease, with thorough disinfection on the
> pupil's return to school, be required of all pupils exposed to an infec-
> tious disease. If such methods are deemed desirable to prevent an
> epidemic in a school, in consequence of one or more of the pupils
> having been exposed to an infectious or contagious disease, why is
> not the principle just as applicable to the prevention of an epidemic
> in a city, in consequence of one or more of the passengers on a vessel
> arriving at that place having been exposed to one of what may be
> considered the epidemic diseases? To ask this question seems to me
> to answer it affirmatively.[71]

The openness of Britain's sanitary zone made possible by the English
System, whether regarded as grounded in the hypocrisy expressed
above or as a reflection of a superior sanitary infrastructure, con-
trasted starkly with the tightening of American borders from the end
of the century. If the English System looked to defend the interests of
trade, United States' quarantine appeared to buttress American
nativism and the increasingly rigorous requirements for entry.[72]
Commerce, critics argued, explained Britain's rejection of quarantine during the cholera epidemic and the willingness to release
potentially infected immigrants into the community. In the United
States the situation was reversed. Economic concerns were seemingly sacrificed to the creation of barriers to the entry of 'infected'
immigrants. The twenty-day quarantine detention period was particularly harmful to trade coming into New York and to the business
of many American steamship companies, but it was successful in

reducing the average number of migrants who arrived into New York each month by up to ninety-three per cent.[73]

In the more agreeable language of public health Americans argued that strict quarantine, although detrimental to the economic interests of maritime trade, was no more damaging to commerce than the label of 'infected port' which would be applied should a contagion be imported:

> It will be admitted by all that the sanitary interests of the United States call for the exclusion, by proper restrictive measures, of all exotic, pestilential diseases; and it can be shown that even from an economic point of view, a single wide-spread epidemic of yellow fever or cholera costs more than our commerce with permanently infected ports is worth.[74]

Whether port health practices were constructed around economic or immigration agendas, scientific medicine, bacteriology and new diagnostic techniques were only employed at the ports when they could reinforce or justify these priorities. During the 1892 epidemic, bacteriological testing was only employed in the United States to prove that cholera had entered the country, thus justifying the use of quarantine. The knowledge derived from bacteriology that the incubation period for cholera was only five to eight days was ignored.[75] As Charles Wilson of the New York Board of Health wrote, 'all that science can do, has been done in the way of preparation should the pest come; all that science can suggest to lessen the evil effects of the pest, should it break out, is either finished or now in the course of completion.'[76] In American, as in British, ports there was a subordination of laboratory medicine to political agendas. In the United States the clear political agenda which selectively employed and ignored the bacterial aetiology of cholera was the nativistic resistance to the immigration of poor European migrants – primarily at this time, Eastern European Jews.

After 1892

With the passing of any immediate threat from cholera after 1892–93, on both sides of the Atlantic other diseases began to replace cholera in perceptions of immigrant contagion. The narratives which redefined certain diseases as 'immigrant diseases' or 'contagions' generally emanated from the United States and were quickly adopted for the same purpose amongst British anti-alienists. By the turn of the century Ellis Island[77] and other facilities for the reception of immigrants in America had implemented systems of inspection which could process up to 5,000 people each day at Ellis Island alone. Easily visible and identifiable diseases associated with poverty and overcrowding such as trachoma, the contagious eye disease and favus, which affected the scalp, were incorporated into immigration law and popular perceptions of the contagious 'nature' of immigrants.[78] Trachoma was especially associated with immigrants from 1897 when the Supervising Surgeon General of the U.S. Marine Hospital Service declared it to be a 'dangerous, contagious disease ... seldom seen except among recent immigrants from the eastern end of the Mediterranean, Polish and Russian Jews'.[79] Subsequently, the identification of trachoma became the most common reason for immigrants to be debarred on medical grounds, constituting an estimated eighty per cent of cases rejected under the classification of 'dangerous and loathsome contagious disease' between 1897 and 1902.[80] Nine out of every ten migrants who were diagnosed with trachoma on arrival were refused entry.[81] The American Public Health Association reported at its Annual Meeting in 1903 that

> the ordinary quarantinable diseases were eliminated by efficient quarantine methods, but certain communicable maladies, classed as loathsome or dangerous contagious diseases, existed among immigrants, and constant vigilance and considerable skill were necessary on the part of medical inspectors of immigrants to detect these cases and separate them from the healthy immigrants. The most important of these diseases, because of its frequency, was trachoma. Of the total number of cases of loathsome or dangerous diseases found in immigrants, 87% were due to trachoma and 10% to favus.[82]

Although trachoma was a highly infectious disease which, if untreated, could result in blindness, it was no more prevalent among immigrants than other infections and much less widespread than tuberculosis, for example. Like TB, trachoma was a disease which was easily transmitted in the overcrowded conditions of steerage accommodation; however, as the development of symptoms occurred around five to twelve days after infection – not much less than the time needed to cross the Atlantic – evidence of the disease was often manifest on arrival. The disease inflamed and reddened the eyes, making them weep and form pustules; it was unavoidably visible. It could be quickly diagnosed among the hundreds of immigrants who lined up for inspection after the arrival of a vessel and thus became branded as the most notorious disease of immigration. While tuberculosis presented a significantly larger and more serious problem, the visibility of trachoma's unsightly symptoms meant that immigrants wore their 'undesirability' on their face. For these reasons trachoma was, what Markel has called, a 'central character' on the 'stage of infectious diseases and immigration.'[83]

American port health controls were perceived in Britain to contribute to the risk of disease in British migrant port towns, particularly after 1892. This idea gathered momentum in the early years of the new century. Yet, before 1897 there was no specific connection made in Britain between immigration, issues of port health and trachoma. Indeed, it was not until the issue of immigration restriction began to be seriously considered by the British government in the first years of the twentieth century that trachoma began to emerge in port papers and related medical articles. In the 1889 Select Committee on Emigration and Immigration[84] for example, evidence regarding the health of migrants referred only to their sanitary condition on arrival into British ports and the generalised idea of their propensity to contagious disease. The annual reports of the Port Medical Officers of Health during the nineteenth century referred to the number of cases of cholera[85] and 'indigenous' diseases such as scarlet fever and measles which arrived on incoming vessels; they did not specifically identify cases of trachoma until the turn of the century. The inclusion of trachoma in British port medical reports coincided with the growing prominence of the campaign to introduce legal restrictions to immigration. Appropriated, as in America, because of its conspicuousness, trachoma became for British immigration restrictionists a corporeal representation of the loathsomeness of steerage class migrants. It also came to represent the style and model of American immigration restriction, so admired by British anti-alienists. As Markel explains, 'the stigma of trachoma became an essential consideration in the East European Jewish immigrant's calculus of migration [to America]' as it 'permeated the experience at almost *every* point along the journey.'[86] This essential element in American 'remote control' was heralded at British ports by US consular or shipping company officials who performed the notorious eye examination on hundreds of migrants at the docks prior to their embarkation for America. The inspections, and the disease they searched for, seemed to underscore the absence of any requirement for similar examinations under British law, particularly as trachoma was understood to be a primary reason why a proportion of migrants were debarred from entering the United States and were returned to or remained in Britain for some time before attempting to enter America.

By the turn of the century, the American stigmatisation of immigrants as a particular source of trachoma had also become an integral part of British perceptions of the immigrant as disease carrier.[87] The Royal Commission on Alien Immigration[88] in 1902–03 took evidence from ophthalmic physicians about the disease. Anti-immigration activists began to target the disease in their literature and newspapers. The popular halfpenny newspaper, the *Daily Mirror*, for instance, ran an article on the 'Alien Scourge – Disease Stricken Immigrants' which highlighted Britain's role as 'dumping ground' for those migrants who had trachoma and were thus medically unfit to enter the United States:

> Recent investigations have shown enormous prevalence of the highly contagious eye disease known as trachoma among recent immigrants.
>
> Trachoma subjects are rigidly barred from entering the United States, where it is admitted that many of the Russian Jews, now transmigrant in London, are bound. At the Royal Ophthalmic Hospital in City Road it was stated that during the last week or so the Russian Jews suffering from incipient or developed trachoma have been flocking for advice and treatment.
>
> On one day, out of 160 new patients, 102 were aliens, mostly with eye disease ... Most of them follow the same formula: 'Can I go to America?' They do not want the treatment so much as expert advice on the possibility of passing the medical examination at the ports of arrival.
>
> Once told that the disease would cause them to be sent back they disappear. They know their forward voyage is impossible, and seem to take no interest in curing the disease.
>
> Thus they remain in the metropolis to become a source of infection for others.[89]

Following America's lead, trachoma and steerage class migrants were conflated in much of the popular and political consciousness about immigration in Britain. Just as cholera had represented the contaminating nature of immigrants in the early 1890s, by the turn of the century trachoma, and to a lesser extent favus, came to represent all that was pernicious in the arrival of migrants in both Britain and America. The trachoma-stricken immigrant not only threatened to spread the contagious microbe which caused the disease, but also embodied a sickness which threatened the integrity of the English

System. Like cholera the disease sat uncomfortably between the neat categorisations of 'exotic' and 'indigenous' which had guided responses to imported infections for most of the previous century. Well-explored and enumerated cases of trachoma among the 'native' urban poor of English cities clearly showed the disease to be 'indigenous', commonly occurring within local communities. Its special identification, however, with a foreign population reoriented its origin to somewhere outside the domestic realm and beyond the bailiwick of the ordinary orderly sanitary environment. Where associated with migrants, the widespread 'indigenous' eye condition transmogrified into something alien and dangerous. What was foreign about the disease became the people with whom it was associated. Migrant-borne trachoma could not be managed, like other 'indigenous' diseases, within the urban and maritime 'English' sanitary zone. Rather, the bodies of 'aliens' and the diseases they carried represented separate and migratory places that precluded integration into the 'domestic' sanitary environment.

Conclusion

By the turn of the century, the English System was well established in the precepts of littoral disease control. Vessels and people from around the world arrived at the ports daily. Quarantine had been abolished and internationally the English System had come to exemplify 'modern' public health practice, or at least had come to be accepted as a viable alternative to quarantine. Yet, two factors in the early 1890s led to marked changes in the operation of the port health system over the next dozen, or so, years. The first, as we have seen, was the cholera epidemic of 1892 and the idea that its source was a particular class of migrant from Eastern and Central Europe. The second was the solutions adopted by the United States to the shared idea that immigrants were the carriers of disease. Britain was certainly affected by the extreme quarantine measures implemented in America in response to the 1892 epidemic and the execution of the 1891 Immigration Act. Yet, as Schloss showed, neither of these had a numerically significant effect on the number of migrants returned from America to Britain. The crucial impact, rather, was how particularly the latter altered British ideas about immigration restriction. America and Britain were linked through the western migration of Europeans and the systems of 'remote control' that helped to define that experience, as well as the eastern movement of those migrants who were expelled from America under ever-tightening definitions of 'desirability' and 'undesirability'. The statistical inconsequence of returned migrants did little to diminish the intensity of this relationship. The identification of trachoma as an immigrant disease in America filtered into British perceptions of, primarily, East European migrants and subsequently to the notice and into the reports of the Port Medical Officers.

The experience of the 1892 cholera epidemic together with subsequent American immigration and quarantine policies heightened awareness in Britain of both the presence of migrants and, perhaps more worrying, transmigrants, and the lack of powers to refuse entry to those deemed 'undesirable'. The assurances of the English System, that the arrival of contagious disease did not pose a risk to the public health if sanitary measures and controls were meticulously administered, was undermined by what *The Lancet* had called 'so many minute migratory fragments of the locality whence [the migrants] came'.[90] The additional anxiety that Britain was becoming the home of 'diseased' migrants not 'good enough' for the United States led to an intensifying revision, from the mid-1890s, of the procedures that governed the arrival of different people and bodies at the ports. Directly and indirectly, then, the policies and practices of American border health stimulated and propelled a transformation in the regulation of British port health from a paradigm focused on the origin of disease to one which converged on the origin of the diseased.

Notes

1   M.J. Landa, *The Alien Problem and Its Remedy* (London: P.S. King & Son, 1911).

2   From Nicholas J. Evans, *Aliens en route: European Transmigration via the UK, 1836–1914* (PhD thesis, University of Hull, 2006).

3   Transmigrants to the United States arrived and departed from London, or arrived into one of the East coast ports (e.g. Hull) and were transported by trains brought right into the port, to departure ports on the West coast (e.g. Liverpool). Not all transmigrants through the United Kingdom were en route to America. Others travelled to Australia, Canada, South Africa and South America. Approximately one third of those Jewish migrants who settled in Australia, for example, had spent enough time in the United Kingdom for them to have learned a small amount of English by the time they arrived in Australia.

S. Rutland, *Edge of the Diaspora – Two Centuries of Jewish Settlement in Australia*, Second Revised Edition (Sydney: Brandl & Schlesinger, 1997), p. 77.

4 Garrard, *The English and Immigration*, p. 24.

5 Aristide Zolberg, 'Matters of State: Theorizing Immigration Policy,' in Charles Hirschman, Philip Kasinitz and Josh De Wind (eds), *The Handbook of International Migration: The American Experience* (New York: Russell Sage, 2000), 71–93.

6 For example: Tobias Brinkmann, '"Travelling with Ballin": The Impact of American Immigration Policies on Jewish Transmigration within Central Europe, 1880–1914,' *International Review of Social History*, 53 (2008), 459–84; Tobias Brinkmann, 'From Immigrants to Supranational Transmigrants and Refugees: Jewish Migrants in New York and Berlin Before and After the Great War,' *Comparative Studies of South Asia, Africa and the Middle East*, 30–1 (2010), 47–57; Gur Alroey, 'Out of the Shtetl. In the Footsteps of Eastern European Jewish Emigrants to America, 1900–1914,' *Leidschrift*, 21–1 (2007), pp. 92–122; Adam McKeown, 'Global Migration, 1846–1940,' *Journal of World History*, 15 (2004), 155–90; and Torsten Feys, 'The Visible Hand of Shipping Interests in American Migration Policies,' *Tijdschrift voor Sociale en Economische Geschiedenis*, 7–1 (2010), 39–62.

7 Aristede Zolberg, 'The Archaeology of "Remote Control",' in Andreas Fahrmeir, Faron, Olivier and Weil, Patrick (eds), *Migration Control in the North Atlantic World: The Evolution of State Practices in Europe and the United States from the French Revolution to the Inter-War Period* (New York: Berghahn Books, 2003), 195–222.

8 See Aristede Zolberg, *A Nation by Design: Immigration Policy in the Fashioning of America* (Cambridge, MA: Harvard University Press, 2006).

9 See, Fairchild, *Science at the Borders*.

10 *Ibid.*, p. 47.

11 *Ibid.*, p. 74.

12 Brinkmann, 'Travelling with Ballin,' p. 469.

13 *Ibid.*, p. 95.

14 *Ibid.*, p. 96.

15 Kraut, *Silent Travelers*, p. 51.

16 Howard-Jones, 'The Scientific Background... 3', p. 370.

17 *National Board of Health Bulletin*, 1, 1 (28 June 1879), p. 2.

18 Goodman, *International Health Organisations*, p. 61.

19 Alison Bashford and Catie Gilchrist, 'The Colonial History of the 1905 Aliens Act,' *The Journal of Imperial and Commonwealth History*, 40, 3 (2012), 409–37.

20 Evidence of Dr. F.A.C.Tyrrell, Medical Officer to the London School Board, and Surgical Officer to the Royal London Ophthalmic Hospital:

Minutes of Evidence Taken Before the Royal Commission on Alien Immigration, 1903, vol. II (London: HMSO, 1903) [Cd. 1742], 3670.

21 LMA, Board of Deputies of British Jews, ACC/3121/B02/01/003.

22 'Report by Mr Schloss: American Legislation and Practice', *Reports to the Board of Trade on Alien Immigration,* 1893 (London: HMSO, 1893), p. 10.

23 *Reports to the Board of Trade on Alien Immigration,* 1893 (London: HMSO, 1893).

24 *Ibid.,* pp. 87–9.

25 Although Schloss's figures are of particular interest, they must be placed within the context of 1892 conditions. These figures might be wholly unrepresentative of other – non-epidemic – years. The regulations put in place in 1892 in response to the cholera epidemic drastically reduced the number of immigrants crossing the Atlantic. The over-all figures for the number of steerage class immigrants arriving into the Port of New York during the 1892 calendar year were down 13% on the previous year, and during the last quarter of 1892 figures were down between 55 and 87% on 1891 figures.

26 Schloss, *On Alien Immigration,* 1893, p. 87.

27 *Ibid.,* p. 87; TABLE II. – (New York); TABLE III. – (New York); and TABLE XVIII. – (All Ports).

28 *Ibid.,* TABLE II. – (New York).

29 *Ibid.,* p. 88.

30 *Ibid.,* p. 88.

31 Krista Maglen, *Investigating the Immigrant Experience: Poor Relief Applications, Computer Analysis and European Immigrants in Glasgow, 1881–1896* (MPhil Dissertation, Glasgow University, 1997–98).

32 SRA D-HEW 17/291 – 81277.

33 Her subsequent fate was not recorded.

34 SRA D-HEW 17/358 – 1073.

35 *BMJ,* 12 Sept. 1896, p. 700.

36 Letter dated 4 Aug. 1896, NA MT9/559/13197.

37 *BMJ,* 10 Sept. 1892, p. 604.

38 *The New York Times,* 29 Aug. 1892, p. 1a.

39 [Circular. 1892. Department No. 150] *Quarantine Restrictions upon Immigration to Aid the Prevention of the Introduction of Cholera into the United States* (Treasury Department, Office of the Supervising Surgeon-General, U.S. Marine Hospital Service, Sept. 1, 1892), *NARA s. exdoc. 52 (52–2) Congressional Series Set, vol. 3056,* also see, *BMJ,* 10 Sept. 1892, p. 606.

40 *Ibid.*

41 Markel, *Quarantine!,* p. 98.

42 *Ibid.,* p. 104. The Medical Officer of the Port of New York, Jenkins, wrote in his 1892 Annual Report that the known incubation period of cholera was two to five days.

43 Members of the Council included T.M. Prudden and Hermann Biggs, who had both studied in Germany under Koch and who both 'played major roles in the introduction of bacteriological research to the United States', Elizabeth Fee and Evelynn Hammonds, 'Science, Politics, and the Art of Persuasion: Promoting the New Scientific Medicine in New York City', Rosner (ed.), *Hives of Sickness*, 155–96, pp. 157–64.

44 *Journal of the American Medical Association*, 22 Oct. 1892, p. 505.

45 Letter from T. Sherman (Consul, Liverpool) to W. Wharton (Assistant Secretary of State, Washington) No. 180, 15 Sept. 1892, NARA, *Consular Correspondence*, Dispatches From Consuls – Liverpool, 1 Jan 1891–1 Dec 1896 (States Department Central Files, Record Group 59, National Archives Microfilm Publication M141, roll T-52), Archives II.

46 *Ibid.*

47 *Ibid.*

48 *Ibid.*

49 Markel, *Quarantine!*, p. 140.

50 Rosenberg, *The Cholera Years*, p. 114.

51 This reduction may also be accounted for in improved sanitary conditions in New York. See Charles Rosenberg, *Explaining Epidemics and Other Studies in the History of Medicine* (Cambridge: Cambridge University Press, 1992), pp. 219–29; and John Duffy, *The Sanitarians: A History of American Public Health* (Chicago: University of Illinois Press, 1990), pp. 177–81.

52 See chapter 3.

53 See Evans, *Death in Hamburg*, pp. 372–9.

54 *BMJ*, 15 Oct. 1892, p. 861.

55 Markel, *Quarantine!*, p. 101.

56 *Ibid.*, p. 115.

57 *The Lancet*, Sept. 17, 1892, p. 672.

58 *Ibid.*

59 Stern, 'Buildings, Boundaries and Blood,' p. 70.

60 Markel, *Quarantine!*, p. 104.

61 *Ibid.*, p. 153.

62 *Ibid.*, p. 170.

63 *Ibid.*, p. 180.

64 *New York Medical Journal*, 1892, vol. 56, p. 355.

65 *Medical News* (Philadelphia), 1892, vol. 61, p. 322.

66 *Ibid.*

67 Thomas P. Hughes, 'Sanitation Versus Quarantine', *North American Review*, 155 (1892), 638.

68 The paper was read before the Section in Public Health of the New York Academy of Medicine, 19 September 1892.

69 *New York Medical Journal*, 1892, vol. 56, p. 355.

70 *Ibid.*

71 *Ibid.*

72 See Markel, *Quarantine!*; Kraut, *Silent Travelers*; and John Higman, *Strangers in the Land: Patterns of American Nativism, 1860–1925* (New Brunswick: Rutgers University Press, 1988).

73 Markel, *Quarantine!*, p. 140.

74 George Sternberg (Major and Surgeon, U.S. Army), 'The Reconciliation of Our Commercial and Sanitary Interests', *Reports on the Sanitation of Ships and Quarantine – Prepared by the Supervising Surgeon-General, U.S. Marine Hospital Service, For the Use of the International American Conference* (Washington: Government Printing Office, 1890), p. 19, *NARA s. exdoc. 58 (51–1), Congressional Serial Set, vol. 2685*.

75 Markel, *Quarantine!*, p. 105; see also, Fee and Hammonds, 'Science, Politics and the Art of Persuasion', pp. 161–2.

76 'Safe-Guards against the Cholera', *North American Review*, 155 (1892), 491.

77 Opened in late 1892.

78 See Birn, 'Six Seconds Per Eyelid'; and Howard Markel, '"The Eyes Have It": Trachoma, the Perception of Disease, the United States Public Health Service, and the American Jewish Immigration Experience, 1897–1924', *Bulletin of the History of Medicine*, 74:3 (2000), 525–60.

79 Markel, 'The Eyes Have It', p. 533.

80 *Ibid.*, p. 535.

81 *Ibid.*, p. 531.

82 *American Medicine* (Philadelphia), 1903, vol. 6, p. 771.

83 Markel, 'The Eyes Have It', p. 528.

84 *Report from the Select Committee on Emigration and Immigration (Foreigners) – Together with Proceedings of the Committee, Minutes of Evidence and Appendix* (London: Hansard, 1889) [311].

85 Only the case of yellow fever on the *Neva* in Southampton, 1889, was reported and plague appeared in the reports from 1899.

86 Markel, 'The Eyes Have It', pp. 528 & 560.

87 Krista Maglen, 'Importing Trachoma: The Introduction into Britain of American Ideas of an 'Immigrant Disease', 1892–1906', *Immigrants and Minorities*, 25, 1 (March 2005), 80–99.

88 See chapter 5.

89 *Daily Mirror*, 6 Dec. 1904, Home Office cutting, NA HO45/ 10303/117267.

90 *The Lancet*, 3 Sept. 1892, p. 592.

5

Aliens in the sanitary zone

In 1896 the old barrier of quarantine finally gave way to the English System with the repeal of the Quarantine Act of 1825, and the practice and administration of port health was no longer divided. Britain's success in averting the spread of cholera in 1892 and the subsequent European acknowledgement that the system of sanitary surveillance had prevented a British epidemic hastened the legal removal of quarantine from the statute books, for all diseases. Yet the question of health at the ports remained open. The increasing belief that migrants were a source of imported infectious disease in Britain – a by-product of the 1892 cholera and reaction to American regulation – encouraged the intensifying momentum against 'alien' immigration and calls for the inclusion in any new immigration legislation of restrictions to the entry of migrants who arrived displaying the signs and symptoms of disease.

The primary focus of the anti-alien debate which developed with particular force in Britain during the first years of the twentieth century was not, however, related to health, but rather the economic consequences of immigration.[1] Those arguing for immigration restriction emphasised the problems of an extended workforce, inadequate housing, and the production and introduction into the market of cheap goods. Overcrowding in immigrant neighbourhoods, primarily in London's East End as well as in Liverpool, Hull, Glasgow and other cities, was frequently described and presented as an illuminating manifestation of the immigrant 'problem'. Yet the health problems which appeared to flourish and be nurtured in the urban slums of port towns were integral to the economic debates of anti-alienism, because they contributed to the wider narrative of migrants as a charge upon the public funds and as drains on the resources of urban, including sanitary, authorities. So, diseases brought into the ports with arriving migrants were seen to both put pressure upon the resources of the sanitary authorities as well as pose a threat to the health of the population. While the link that had been established between immigration and disease was an important part of the anti-alien debate and found a place within the legislation resulting from it, it did not occupy as central a place in anti-alien concerns over immigration or excite the same fervour or vivid imagery as it did in the United States. Nor was it considered by many to be a problem requiring legal intervention. Throughout the debates leading up to Britain's new immigration legislation – the Aliens Act 1905 – the Port Sanitary Authorities fiercely defended the ability of current structures to sufficiently prevent the introduction and spread of infectious disease and their complete control over diseased vessels and individuals arriving into British ports, so recently acquired from the Customs Service.

This final chapter will examine how those arguing for immigration restriction used the issue of disease; how the example of American policy and practice played an important role in this part of the debate; and why ultimately, despite the rhetoric and new categorisations, infectious disease did not occupy the same place on the centre stage of anti-alien activity as in the United States. The Port Medical Officers of Health, and those involved with their work were among the first to encounter the migrants when they arrived in Britain. The concerns they voiced among themselves about the threat of infection accompanying migrant vessels remained evident after 1892 and into the new century, but when giving evidence to the Royal Commission on Alien Immigration in 1902–03 and in official testimony relating to immigration legislation, these officers assured the relevant authorities that the risk was minimal. They maintained confidence in the English System and in the competency of supporting inland sanitary structures and systems to deal adequately with any risk. The primary concern of the Medical Officers was ensuring that migrants remained within these systems and under the observation of the sanitary authorities. Crucial to this sanitary surveillance was the acquisition of information about migrants' identity and intended destinations when they arrived at the ports. Between 1892 and 1905 this was the sole means of managing and overseeing immigration, and the Port Sanitary Authorities had staked an important claim to it.

The abolition of quarantine

During the years 1892–95 the Port Sanitary Authorities retained the powers granted under the Local Government Board General Cholera Orders during the 1892 epidemic. These Orders included additions to their powers and an extension to their jurisdiction with regard to cases of cholera. The rigorous investigation of passengers' forward addresses (which will be discussed later in this chapter) was continued. However, once the threat of cholera had again retreated, the special authority of the General Orders was removed and power to deal with cases of cholera, along with yellow fever and plague, was once again placed within the jurisdiction of the Customs Service.

From late 1893 the immediate danger of cholera had passed, and serious discussion finally began in the Houses of Parliament regarding the abolition of quarantine. However, the old concerns remained, particularly in relation to the implications for trade of removing the legal 'safety-net' of quarantine. Departments, including the Board of Trade, Local Government Board and Treasury Chambers, exchanged anxious notes to check and double-check that no harm could befall British foreign trade if the Quarantine Act was removed. Despite confidence in the English System, there remained a serious concern that difficulties might await British vessels when 'they go to countries which believe in quarantine'.[2] However, the Board of Trade and Foreign Office gave assurances that these concerns were unfounded.[3] With these, the Public Health Act 1896[4] quickly passed with ease through both Houses of Parliament and 'the remarkable anomaly of one disease being dealt with by one Authority and another by a second Authority at the same time and under the same conditions'[5] was brought to an end. The Act came into force on 7 November 1896 and applied to the whole of the United Kingdom. Primarily, it transferred all the authority previously held by the Privy Council and Customs Service over ships arriving with cholera, yellow fever and plague to the Local Government Board and Port Sanitary Authorities. These particular powers – to inspect and detain an entire ship with suspected as well as actual cases – only applied to the three traditionally quarantinable diseases, however, and did not extend to 'indigenous' diseases. Thus, the capabilities of the Port Sanitary Authorities were only expanded in relation to the former and not the latter.[6]

The Act extended the definition of an 'infected' vessel, and therefore the ability to inspect and detain, to include cases of 'exotic' disease which occurred on board, up to and including departure from its last port, rather than 'after it had left'. It also included two new provisions. The first reinforced the expertise of the ship's surgeon, ensuring a completion of the professionalization of port medicine, making medical men solely qualified to identify the presence of disease at the littoral. As the Port of London Sanitary Committee described, it

> requires [the surgeon] to give a responsible professional certificate as to whether there has been any case on board. The Master's certificate was, strictly speaking, of no value, as he certified to a matter of which he had no expert knowledge, whereas a Medical Certificate is of a known and definite worth.[7]

The second provision gave power to the Port Medical Officer to require the master of a vessel to bring his ship 'to' or to moor or anchor the vessel in a place convenient for undertaking a thorough medical inspection. This remedied a weak element in the previous law which called on the master of a vessel to *permit* his vessel to be boarded and examined.[8] Furthermore, 'as to the necessity for detention, and of the length of such detention, the Medical Officer of Health [was] the sole judge'.[9]

Thus, after more than half a century of serious endeavour to do away with the burdensome and exorbitant obligations of quarantine, the system was finally removed from the statute books and the Local Government Board and its Medical Officers were alone responsible for the health of British ports. Only four years later the newly expanded English System was tested against one of the previously quarantinable diseases – plague – during the pandemic of 1899–1900. Arriving first in Glasgow in August 1900,[10] it visited numerous cities around England and Wales. Customs Officers still boarded vessels under the Customs Consolidations Act of 1876 which regulated the importation of goods. Although they no longer had any jurisdiction over the health of ships, during the threatened and actual arrival of plague in 1899–1900 Customs Officers were instructed to assist the Medical Officers of Health in all matters relating to inspection and to ensure that the Port Sanitary Authorities were aware at all times of the arrival of vessels from infected ports. The Port Sanitary Authorities enforced isolation of the sick and sanitary surveillance of healthy passengers from infected vessels both at and away from the port in much the same way it had during the 1892 cholera epidemic. It was the first time plague had been dealt with by anything other than quarantine, allowing healthy contacts to enter into the community under the surveillance of health officers, isolating only those individuals who suffered from and exhibited symptoms. There was no separation of the population from personal or sea spaces linked by plague, permitting, finally, the realisation of an unobstructed sanitary zone that provided protection while maintaining ample liberalism in the regular activities of the ports.

In addition to this, there were a number of differences between the arrival of plague and that of cholera eight years earlier. Notably, by 1900 bacteriological testing had been incorporated into port health protocol and was used to confirm or deny the existence of plague in suspicious cases. In England and Wales four cases of plague – two in London, one in Liverpool, and the other at 'the Tyne port' – were confirmed by bacteriological testing.[11] In Glasgow thirty-six cases were confirmed in the laboratory. This reflected the general acceptance of bacteriological science that had been reached by the turn of the century and, perhaps, its significantly decreased importance in the politics of port health and imperial maritime connections after the abolition of quarantine.

Yet, although quarantine no longer played a role in British ports, it was still imposed in most other places around the world. Under the convention drawn up at the Venice International Sanitary Conference of 1897, Glasgow was declared to be an infected port. This meant that although sanitary precautions, rather than quarantine, could be used in British ports, foreign ports could impose quarantine on any vessel which had sailed from Glasgow, because plague remained a 'quarantinable' disease. However, the classification of Glasgow as an infected port lasted only until October, and the city was congratulated for its victory over the threatened epidemic through the combined efforts of the sanitary authorities. Experts from around the world had descended on the city to observe the disease and examine how the English System operated in preventing the extension of the disease, and all proclaimed it a great success.[12]

The effective management of plague in 1900 through cooperation between port and local sanitary authorities was based on the same methods of observation as used during the cholera epidemic of 1892. Healthy people were placed under sanitary surveillance in domestic settings away from the port and infected individuals were isolated. However, none of this was aimed primarily at migrants. Unlike in 1892, the focus of prevention was on the arrival of 'suspected' vessels from 'infected' ports, rather than on a specific group or class of people. In Britain, unlike in San Francisco or Sydney for example, the spread of plague was not associated with migrants, nor was it thought to follow particular migration routes.[13] The prevention of cholera, on the other hand, became so directly associated with migrants that it not only relied upon the sanitary authorities, but also depended (as we shall see) upon other organisations to ensure continuous surveillance and control of the people who were perceived to embody it. So, while the plague epidemic highlighted the features and victory of sanitary practices at the ports *par excellence*, cholera, and other diseases which came to be specifically associated with migrants, strained uneasily at the ideals of the English System.

'The duty of keeping these aliens under supervision...'[14]

Central to the problematic relationship between arriving migrants and the English System, highlighted by cholera, was the issue of surveillance. Despite intensifying anxiety about migrants since the cholera epidemic, the only apparatus for managing them until the passing of the Aliens Act in 1905 was the Local Government Board Cholera Order of 1892. It was, as a number of American journals highlighted, the only means of immigration control. Migrants who were unable to provide addresses that could be verified by the local sanitary authorities for surveillance could be detained at the ports and in rare cases were returned to Continental Europe.

For a variety of reasons, however, the ability or willingness of migrants to furnish accurate information to port officials was not always straightforward. The majority of Eastern European migrants were destined for America, and many had booked their passage with agents who organised the various stages of their journey from their places of origin to the United States. These agencies often had offices at the European departure ports of Hamburg, Bremen or Rotterdam, for example, as well as in the transmigration towns of Britain, such as London and Hull. Yet, some were less scrupulous than others, and exploited the naiveté and desperation of many of the migrants. Agents in Europe often sold tickets only as far as London, where migrants were instructed to collect onward tickets from local agency offices. But the London addresses provided by dishonest agents in Europe were often fictional. As a result some migrants arrived with nowhere to stay and had no way of completing the journey they had paid for to America. Questionable agents who did provide temporary accommodation in

London or Hull offered only the most wretchedly overcrowded and unsanitary lodging houses. Port Medical Officers were wary of agency addresses for these reasons and many migrants subsequently found themselves unable to land. With no other connections in Britain, nor funds to find alternative lodgings, these migrants were likely to be detained or rejected by the sanitary authorities, or became susceptible to those looking to exploit their consequent vulnerability.

Recognising the defencelessness of arriving migrants, various groups, particularly in London, gathered at the 'landing places of the riverside' anxious to take advantage of the bewildered arrivals. In his memoirs Abraham Mundy, who was Secretary of the Poor Jews' Temporary Shelter between 1897 and 1946, recalled and described the chief offenders:

> crimps of the worst type were abounding at every landing place, who took charge of the emigrants, presumably to conduct them with their baggage to friends or lodgings. They were, however, in many instances taken to undesirable lodging houses where they were robbed of all their belongings, whilst their young women-folk were decoyed to places of ill repute and shame.[15]

Other kinds of perils also awaited the Jewish arrivals:

> The watchful eyes of the missionaries propagating Christianity amongst the Jews were mainly focused on these people, who they were anxious to ensnare... These 'soul-snatchers' were usually lying in wait at the landing places of the riverside, and on the disembarkation of each load of immigrants from the Continent, they poured upon them and distributed their religious tracts and insidious literature amongst them, inviting them at the same time to their centres to listen to their religious services and preaching, and offering them as a bait assistance in kind.[16]

The Poor Jews' Temporary Shelter was established in October 1885 in Leman Street, Whitechapel, to address this problem and to provide immediate aid to poor immigrants and transmigrants in London.[17] Recognising the 'gatekeeping' function that was beginning to inform the work of the Port Sanitary Authority in London, the Shelter signed an agreement with it in 1893 which allowed their organisation to provide alternative lodging for migrants whose agent had placed them in fictional or notoriously unsanitary accommodation. The agreement originated after the 1892 epidemic at the Port Sanitary Authority's initiation. Collingridge saw such an arrangement as the only way to reduce the costly and time-consuming work created by the increasing number of migrants who were arriving with 'unreliable' addresses. Thus, a deal was negotiated whereby the Shelter would ensure the whereabouts of all Jewish immigrants in London for seven days after arrival on condition that Collingridge promised 'to do his best' to hand over all immigrants to the Shelter, making sure that they 'especially not to be handed over to missionaries or other irresponsible persons'.[18] The agreement also stated that it was the right of the Port Medical Officer to detain any immigrant arriving into the Port of London. Nonetheless, keeping open the space which connected the port with urban environments, Jewish people with questionable addresses were no longer to be detained at the port but handed over to an officer of the Shelter with a 'nominal roll' drawn up by the Port Medical Officer. These migrants were taken to the Shelter where a further 'roll' was taken of their names and their intended addresses which were subsequently examined by officers of the Shelter. Once the Shelter verified their addresses, an officer of the Shelter personally escorted the migrants to the residence. The 'roll', as well as details of anyone who left the Shelter to board another vessel within the period of surveillance (seven days), was forwarded to the Port Sanitary Office at Greenwich. In return, the Port Sanitary Office agreed to furnish the Shelter with a list of all immigrant vessels due to arrive into London, so that they could ensure the presence of a Shelter officer at the riverside.[19] By placing migrants with questionable addresses in the care of the Shelter, the Port Sanitary Authority relieved itself, and local sanitary authorities, from the arduous responsibility of visiting each problematic address and making enquiries about each anticipated guest as well as the conditions of the accommodation.[20] Furthermore, the agreement provided a safeguard in those cases where addresses were found not to be *bona fide*. Rather than having to enforce a costly detention or expulsion, and undermine the openness of the sanitary zone, surveillance of the migrants could be guaranteed at the Shelter until the prescribed time had elapsed.

The arrangement did not always operate smoothly however. The Port Sanitary Authority was disappointed with the frequent 'disappearance' of migrants placed within the care of the Shelter within the seven-day period, while the Shelter complained that a lack of Port Sanitary Authority vigilance was allowing 'the Missionaries to entice away a number of Jewish new arrivals, to unknown addresses, making it difficult for the Shelter and the authorities to trace them'.[21] In February 1894 the Port Sanitary Committee made an official complaint to the Local Government Board stating that they were 'not satisfied from information which [had] reached them that proper care [was] taken by the Committee of the Poor Jews' Temporary Shelter to carry out on their part of the agreement which was entered into.'[22] Collingridge and his colleagues worried that migrants were 'disappearing' on the way from the port to Whitechapel and that the Shelter was not properly inspecting and verifying migrant residences, personally escorting them to the addresses, or returning to the Port Sanitary Office complete and accurate registers of all the migrants placed in their care.[23] In response to these concerns, the Local Government Board convened a conference with Medical Officers of the Port of London and the Whitechapel Sanitary Authorities as well as the President of the Jewish Board of Guardians and organising members of the Shelter.[24] Under some pressure from the Medical Officers, the Shelter agreed that they alone had not properly carried out their part of the original agreement, while stating that the Port Sanitary Authority had been consistent in honouring their side of the agreement. With the Shelter having taken responsibility for the problems which occurred, a new agreement was signed which barely differed from the original except for the inclusion of a further article requiring that the name of the vessel on which migrants arrived be registered on the 'roll'. This way it would be easier to trace individuals from the same vessel should it later be discovered to be infected. It also strengthened the connection between the ports and urban areas, creating a nexus between ships in their maritime environment and the houses, neighbourhoods and local organisations that accommodated newly arrived migrants.

The agreement terminated in 1895 when the General Order of 1892, which specified the medical inspection and registration of all immigrants, was withdrawn because the importation of cholera was no longer deemed to pose a threat. However, although not officially continued, Collingridge and the Shelter's Executive Committee agreed to continue the arrangement on an unofficial and less stringent basis as it had proven to be so mutually beneficial.[25] Yet, with the end of the threat of cholera and the Order removed, the Port Sanitary Authorities retained no specific authority over the arrival of immigrants as distinct from other passenger arrivals.

The General Order focused on the arrival of migrants because they were considered to pose a particular threat during the cholera epidemic. As the English System was based primarily on the principle of observation after disembarkation, the public health threat which resulted from the disappearance of passengers from an infected vessel was great. If possible sources of infection disappeared from view, it became extremely difficult to maintain control over the spread of infection. Distrustful and resourceful migrants gave, for a variety of reasons, false information to the authorities. The false names, plans and destinations not only, as we shall see, drastically distorted immigrant statistics, giving fuel to the anti-alien campaign, but also meant that the sanitary authorities could not monitor the health of migrants who travelled from an infected port for the prescribed seven-day surveillance period. Not knowing where migrants were in the days after disembarkation from an infected, or suspected vessel, meant that an infection could spread before local medical officers could identify and isolate cases where they occurred. It also severed the crucial connection between port and urban sanitary districts. This reticence among migrants to provide correct information about their intended whereabouts fostered the belief among sanitary workers that migrants were particularly 'untrustworthy' and therefore a particular threat to the integrity of the sanitary zone. Migrants were considered especially likely to disappear after disembarkation. This seriously undermined the English System and although responses to arriving migrants were heavily informed by prejudice, there was also an important public health rationale for ensuring the registration of people from infected vessels in this way. It was equally important to Jewish organisations, such as the Poor Jews' Temporary Shelter, that Jewish migrants presented, and were perceived to present, no risk to the public health. In this matter (as in other issues relating to East European immigration and transmigration in Britain) Jewish organisations wished to prevent migrants from provoking any complaints which might potentially excite an anti-Semitic backlash; they also did not wish to see their co-religionists fall into the hands of the 'crimps' and 'missionaries' readily awaiting their arrival. Thus the General Order, while singling out the migrants, encouraged a system for representatives of Jewish organisations to be present in a semi-official capacity alongside the Port Medical Officers at the moment the migrants arrived.

The relationship was mutually advantageous. As well as protecting newly arrived migrants, the Poor Jews' Temporary Shelter and other Jewish organisations, such as the Board of Deputies of British Jews, were often able to obtain more accurate information from the migrants with regard to their intentions. Many of the migrants were anxious about the uniformed Medical Officers and various other officials they encountered at different stages of their journey. Stories and fragmented anecdotes filtered through the waves of migrants moving Westward about what might happen if 'this or that' piece of information was given to the authorities; experience had shown that it was often more prudent to conceal the truth. Migrants frequently lied about the amount of money they possessed, for example, 'because in Russia, if he told an official he had money, the official would have it'.[26] However, the representatives of Jewish organisations posed no such threat and were thus able to acquire more accurate information which they then shared with the Port Sanitary Authorities and the Board of Trade. Even so, despite the advantages Jewish organisations had over sanitary authorities and Board of Trade in obtaining information, migrants continued to 'disappear' and migration statistics remained drastically distorted.

These statistics had a particular bearing on the development of anti-alien sentiment within government circles. Popular discontent about the presence of immigrants in towns and cities such as London, Liverpool, Hull and Grimsby chiefly focused upon the perceived economic privations created by an extended workforce, overcrowding in working class urban neighbourhoods and the idea that immigrants produced goods which undercut the prices of goods produced by native manufacturers.[27] Ultimately, however, it was the number of migrants perceived to be 'swarming' into the country which spearheaded changes to the law with regard to the regulation of immigration. Attempts were made in 1894, 1896 and 1897 to pass legislation against the growing number of immigrants. Yet, Bills drawn up in 1894 and 1897 went no further than one or two readings, with campaigners such as Lord Salisbury unable to gain sufficient support for legislation. Britain's legal and moral traditions which spoke of ideals of liberty of movement and of asylum and which were championed by Liberal politicians hampered the support the Bills needed in Parliament at the early stages of debate. Legal discussions were frequent and difficult, as an article in the *Law Quarterly Review* titled 'Alien Legislation and the Prerogative of the Crown' demonstrated in 1897:

> from a legal and historical point of view the most interesting issue raised is whether or not the Crown, acting for the public welfare, possesses an inherent right, apart from legislation, to exclude or expel aliens whose presence it considers objectionable on public grounds...

There are doubtless groups of persons with strong opinions on moral, scientific, and trade questions, who would collectively furnish reasons for the exclusion of almost every kind of alien, but in dealing with legislation which affects the liberties of foreigners, if we desire to maintain a reputation for liberality and common sense, we must act on such grounds as will be generally recognised as common sense.[28]

However, by 1898 the desire to place restrictions on the number and type of immigrants allowed to enter Britain was beginning to gain political momentum. A Bill which called for the exclusion of anyone deemed to be 'an idiot, insane, pauper', likely to become a public charge, having symptoms of a loathsome or contagious disease, or 'a danger to good order',[29] entered Parliament and was carried through to the final reading of the House of Lords before being discarded. What enabled the Bill to get further than any previous attempt was the strong arguments made by the Earl of Hardwicke and his supporters during the second reading of the Bill in the House of Lords. Hardwicke argued that 'the stream of alien immigration which struck the noble marquis [of Salisbury] as so dangerous in 1894 had increased in volume'.[30]

The Board of Trade, under the authority of the 1836 Aliens Registration Act,[31] collected official statistics relating to immigration into Britain – which included both immigrants and transmigrants. The Act did not place any restrictions on entry, but rather was concerned solely with registration. It had fallen out of use but was revived in 1890 on the recommendation of the 1889 House of Commons Select Committee on Immigration and Emigration. The Committee was not prepared to recommend restrictive immigration legislation at that time but 'contemplate[d] the possibility of such legislation becoming necessary in the future', and felt that it would be necessary to 'ascertain with greater accuracy, and more frequently than the decennial census provides, the number of aliens that remain in this country'.[32] The resulting data collected by the Board of Trade was considered an important indication of the number of migrants who arrived in and departed from Britain and was considered more accurate and up to date than the census. Yet problems which were encountered during the collection of these statistics were problems that also had a particular bearing on the sanitary authorities. Where migrants were lost statistically, they were also lost to sanitary surveillance.

The master of each vessel which arrived in a port where 'Alien Lists' were collected[33] was required to submit a list of all 'aliens' on board.

According to the statute he was obliged to include 'Christian' name, surname, profession, sex, and native country.[34] An officer of the Customs Service who counted the aliens and checked the details recorded by the master verified this information in around one in ten cases.[35] Amongst this information, perhaps the most important statistic, and the issue that became most problematic, represented those migrants who were 'stated to be en route'. This data was crucial because it formed the basis of the Board of Trade statistics – so important in the immigration debate – that indicated the number of aliens who remained in Britain and the number who were destined to travel on to America or another country (that is, those who entered Britain on a strictly temporary basis). The number of migrants 'en route' and the number remaining were determined by those alien passengers who, on arrival, could produce 'through' tickets to places beyond Britain and those who could not. Those who could were 'stated to be en route' and those who could not were 'not stated to be en route' and were thus identified as true immigrants. As the Deputy Comptroller-General of the Board of Trade declared in evidence to the Royal Commission on Alien Immigration, the production of a 'through' ticket was the sole method used to determine these figures because 'there is no such thing as a statistic of intention. There must be some fact to go by'.[36] Thus only those who could produce the necessary ticket were recorded as transmigrant while every other migrant who disembarked at a British port was recorded as an immigrant intent on remaining in Britain.

However, this data was highly problematic. Firstly, the statistics did not account for those migrants who had arranged with their agents to collect an onward ticket from a correspondent in Britain; and secondly, as steamship tickets bore no identification of ownership, they could be exchanged and used for the purposes of the Alien List more than once.[37]

Yet, the patterns which emerge from the statistics clearly demonstrate that tickets determined figures in the Aliens List. The Northern ports of Hull, Grimsby and Leith generally accommodated the 'package' passages of steamship companies which worked in association with the railways in transporting migrants across Britain to West coast ports where vessels were waiting to sail across the Atlantic. Passengers who arrived in these Northern ports usually possessed a ticket paid through to the United States for which Britain was only part of a larger single journey.[38] Data collected in these ports was therefore more straightforward, with the majority being reliably 'stated to be en route'. Such transmigration 'packages' were rarely available through London however, and thus smaller numbers arrived in London who could be recorded as 'stated to be en route'. In 1895, for example, the Board of Trade recorded 13,413 aliens who arrived into London as 'not stated to be en route' and only 141 as 'stated to be en route'. In contrast 2,289 were 'not stated to be en route' in Hull and 23,376 displayed the through tickets which classified them as 'en route'. Similarly in 1902, London recorded 33,046 'not stated to be en route' and only fourteen 'en route', while Hull reported 2,540 and 70,082 respectively.[39] The Board of Trade were aware, however, that some migrants statistically recorded in London as 'not stated to be en route' did actually leave Britain shortly after arrival, and it was in these numbers that problems arose.[40]

The distortion of figures relating to London was precipitated by the actions of the steamship companies. During the second half of the 1890s[41] nine of the major trans-Atlantic shipping companies – Allan Line, Allan State Line, American Line (Liverpool – Philadelphia), American Line (Southampton – New York), Anchor Line, Beaver Line, Cunard Line, Dominion Line and the White Star Line –[42] agreed a minimum fare scale for passage to the United States from the Continent. The arrangement, called the North Atlantic Conference (NAC), had the purpose of halting competitive pricing 'with a view to raising the fares, which at one time sunk down to about 26s'.[43] The agreement ensured all profits made from trans-Atlantic steerage class tickets from the Continent were pooled and divided among the constituent companies and set two levels of pricing. At the end of 1898, the price of a steerage class journey from the Continent to the United States was fixed at £7 15s for Europeans travelling to the United States, while tickets purchased in London for passage to the United States cost £5 16s. This fare was only available to purchase in Britain and was restricted to British residents. However, the difference allowed a potential saving of around £2.[44] The same was true in 1903 when evidence was taken at the Royal Commission on Alien Immigration. By then the price for a voyage from a Continental to an American port was £8 10s, while the price for a ticket from London was only £5 10s.[45] The disparity in fares was significant and made the purchase of tickets in Britain very attractive to poor migrants, even factoring in the cost of crossing from Hamburg or Bremen to London, which was only 15s to 24s. Such a saving would have made a considerable difference in the lives of most steerage passengers, but also made a considerable contribution to the profits of the

NAC on Continental passengers. In order to protect these profits, therefore, and ensure that migrants did not cross the Channel to buy the cheaper ticket, the NAC stipulated that only people who had been resident in Britain for at least five weeks could purchase the more economical fare and voyage from Britain to America. As far as the NAC was concerned, this period officially constituted British residency and classified a migrant as an 'English passenger'.

Hardly foolproof, the system allowed significant space for fraud to take place among those looking to secure the cheaper fare. Emigration agents operating in Europe sold migrants tickets to London and advised them to declare that Britain was their intended destination. This information, and the lack of an onward ticket, was then entered with their names and nationalities in the Board of Trade's Alien List as 'not stated to be en route'. Agents advised migrants, after leaving the port, to then temporarily change their names, declare that they had been resident in Britain for any period over five weeks and then purchase tickets from the agent's correspondent in Britain which would take them from London or another British departure port to the United States. These migrants would have been registered on the Aliens List as immigrating into Britain. However, within a few hours or days they would depart for the United States under a different name, stating that they had been resident in Britain for over five weeks, and indeed often stating periods of up to two years.[46] Consequently, as the Board of Deputies and the Poor Jews' Temporary Shelter argued, the figures recorded by the Board of Trade on the Aliens List, and used by those wishing to impose restrictions on immigration to demonstrate the 'alarming' and increasing number of immigrants arriving into Britain every year, grossly misrepresented the number of migrants who entered the country and stayed.

The Board of Trade attempted to compensate for the discrepancies caused by migrants' manipulation of NAC price structures. They compiled yearly statistics relating to the number of migrants whose name was noticed to occur both on the Alien List and on lists compiled of departing emigrants (Table 5.1).

However, the number of migrants 'ascertained to be *en route* in addition to the Aliens List' only represented those migrants whose names were noticed on departure to correspond with those recorded on the arrivals list. As these migrants had not chosen to change their names, they probably departed for the United States on one of the few non-NAC

Table 5.1 Aliens stated and not stated to be en route, 1893–1902[47]

Year	Not stated to be en route	Stated to be en route	Ascertained to be en route in addition to aliens list
1893	31,056	79,518	420
1894	28,682	35,512	2,166
1895	30,528	44,637	2,074
1896	35,448	40,036	2,961
1897	38,851	32,221	2,676
1898	40,785	32,177	2,336
1899	50,884	49,947	2,889
1900	62,505	71,682	3,972
1901	55,464	79,140	3,879
1902	66,471	118,478	7,964[a]

[a] Provisional figure, subject to slight amendment.

vessels which sold steerage tickets to European migrants from British ports. Because of the conditions imposed by the NAC, few who purchased an onward ticket to the United States within five weeks would not have changed their names. The figures represented in the table above, then, only represent migrants who kept their name and who happened to be recognised by a Customs Officer on departure. No systematic cross-referencing took place:

> We do not attempt to trace the correspondence of names until the officer of Customs has stated that he has reason to believe them to be going on. We never attempt to compare the alien list as a whole with the passenger outward list as a whole. We should probably find a great many more correspondences if we did.[48]

In 1902, for example, the twelve per cent of migrants who were initially 'not stated to be en route', and who were later recorded by the Board of Trade to have departed for 'other countries', probably represented only a very small percentage of those who actually departed, as the majority hid their identity in order to escape having to pay for the more expensive Continental fare.

The Board of Deputies of British Jews and the Poor Jews' Temporary Shelter were aware of the methods migrants engaged in in order to obtain a less costly ticket to America. Similarly aware of how these methods distorted official statistics relating to the number of immigrants who remained in Britain, both organisations wrote to the Board of Trade to try to draw attention to the inaccuracies. However, their calculations were only based on approximations and figures they derived from the Board of Trade. In addition, the alternative figures they provided related, or attempted to relate, specifically to East European Jews. Religion was not recorded by the Board of Trade and nationality was the only indication of religious affiliation. Russian or Polish 'Hebrew' was, however, often used. It is thus difficult to determine the accuracy of these organisations' figures as nationality was also not always analysed separately in the statistics produced by the Board of Trade.[49] Thus the figure they estimated of 1,700, thought to be the number of migrants who remained in England [sic] in 1898 in excess of 'foreigners' recorded to have left, is impossible to verify. The Poor Jews' Temporary Shelter insisted that although this might be an accurate figure for the number of East Europeans recorded to have remained, they argued that because an estimated 30,000 migrants departed England registered under false names, and as such as 'English residents', there was an actual deficit of 28,300 migrants for the year 1898, rather than a 1,700 increase.[50] Yet it was also impossible to know, they argued, of more than one case in ten and the numbers represented by the Board of Trade were even more misleading than had been initially apparent: 'The result [of the "fraud"] is most serious and makes the Board of Trade Returns of the number of foreigners leaving England absolutely inaccurate'.[51]

The distortion of immigrant statistics was the primary and most important consequence of this contravention of NAC pricing. The resulting data were brandished by the anti-alien campaign to demonstrate the extent of the 'influx' and were a substantial piece of evidence used against unrestricted immigration. Another consequence of the 'fraud', however, was that the sanitary authorities were less able to maintain their necessary surveillance over migrants. When migrants presented false names and destinations they undermined the ability of sanitary authorities to monitor passengers from infected ports or vessels. However, the 'disappearance' of the migrants was a response not to the requirements of the sanitary system but to the fixed pricing of the NAC on passage from the Continent to the United States.[52] Either way, the results were significant for the underlying assumption of anti-alienists that immigrants were 'swamping' Britain, and the secondary notion that Jewish immigrants in particular could not be contained and controlled with the protective apparatus of the English System.

The Royal Commission on Alien Immigration

Although the issue of immigration restriction was not new, it only began to gain political traction after 1900 when a vocal group of Conservatives won seats in London's East End campaigning on anti-alienism. The new Member for Stepney, Major William Evans-Gordon, led the movement toward restriction and, as well as pushing the issue within the House, founded what Paul Knepper has called 'the first quasi-fascist organisation in Britain', the British Brothers' League (BBL).[53] Allied with the Londoners' League (LL), formed at a meeting of the East London Conservative Association in 1901, the two organisations provided a link between popular anti-alien discontent and the government. Closely linked to the Conservative Party through their leadership, both groups used their influence to lobby Parliament for the introduction of restrictive immigration legislation.[54]

Central to Conservative anti-alien rhetoric was the language of national efficiency, which saw the unrestricted immigration of 'physically enfeebled', pauper aliens, as damaging to the health and strength of the 'national stock'.[55] These ideas were conflated with concerns about the poor physical condition of British troops in the South African war and the perceived challenges to Britain's imperial dominance brought about by the degeneration of the working (fighting) classes. The arrival of thousands of poor Jewish immigrants was presented as compounding these problems, particularly, as David Feldman argues, within a context where Britain's key imperial competitors, Germany and the United States, had put in place immigration legislation.[56] While the issue of immigration restriction could therefore cross party lines and class, as its foundations were rooted in ideas of 'home and country', it was dominated by Conservatives and found little support among Liberals. Non-parliamentary individuals within the leadership of the BBL and LL, such as J.L. Silver and William Stanley Shaw, objected to the political aim of using the issue of immigration to increase Conservative Party membership and support and its resulting threat of pushing East End politics in a more radical direction. Shaw, the first president of the BBL, claimed that the 'politicians refused to support me unless I became a tool in their hands', which resulted in his resignation.[57]

However, the appeal of the organisations clearly demonstrated the importance of the issue in East End politics. At its first annual general meeting the BBL claimed to have a membership of 12,000, and by 1902 was able to amass 45,000 signatures on a petition supporting its demands. Two massive public meetings of over 4000 people at the Peoples' Palace, the first in January 1902 under the auspices of the BBL and then in November 1903 under the LL, demonstrated the growing popular support in London for the restriction of immigration. Strengthening the link between East End anti-alienists and Westminster, the BBL formed ties with the Parliamentary Pauper Immigration Committee which was formed in August 1901 and headed by Conservative Sheffield MP, Howard Vincent. Drawing on the increasing pressure of popular activity in the East End, Conservatives such as Evans-Gordon and S.F. Ridley (Bethnal Green) used these relationships and asserted pressure in Parliament for reform. A deputation of the LL, for example, met with the Home Secretary, the President of the Board of Trade and the President of the Local Government Board, in 1901, impressing on them the 'urgent need of legislation with reference to overcrowding in South and East London and to the constantly increasing influx of pauper aliens.'[58] Evans-Gordon, together with two other Conservative Members of Parliament, presented the demands of the League which received a sympathetic hearing and assurances that the matter would be supported and presented to both Cabinet and at the next Session of Parliament.

However, in January 1902 Evans-Gordon expressed in a speech in the House of Commons great disappointment that no mention of alien immigration had been made in the King's speech at the opening of Parliament. He emphasised that alien immigration had become a prominent and 'urgent' issue which required 'legislation to regulate and restrict the immigration of destitute aliens into London and other cities in the United Kingdom.'[59] As MP for Stepney, he pressed the issue of overcrowding and unemployment, but he also stressed that as 'the American law was going to be strengthened ... it was a mathematical certainty ... that the flow must go down the channels that were open. There was only one channel really open now, and that was the channel which led to these shores.'[60] He argued that the desire to regulate was based entirely on 'social and economic grounds', and that any claims that anti-alien movements were motivated by anti-Semitism was unfounded:

> I know it has been said by some people that this is a racial question, and that we are trying to stir up anti-Semitic feeling. I will not detain the House going into such a question. The reverse is the fact. No one deplores more than I do the attitude taken up by some foreign countries towards the Jews...

> It is unfortunate that the racial question should be introduced into the matter, but it is difficult for us to enlighten the uneducated classes of this country upon the subject. All they know is that they are being turned out of their homes and the neighbourhoods in which they are obliged to live, in order to carry on their work, and that their places are being taken by Russian and Polish Jews, and you cannot persuade them that it is not a racial question. They naturally take a hatred to the Jewish people. It is for the Government to prevent that anti-Semitic feeling which, if something is not done to check the influx of aliens into this country, must inevitably result in an outbreak of very grave proportions.[61]

Arguing that the Anglo-Jewish community shared his beliefs and supported his call for restriction as an attempt to stem the 'grave risk of an anti-Semitic colour being imparted to this controversy' Evans-Gordon tried to distance himself from accusations of anti-Semitism.[62] However, despite his claims to the contrary, he frequently employed anti-Semitic imagery and quickly descended into bigotry. In explaining to the House of Commons, for example, why it was important to introduce national immigration legislation when the problems encountered with the immigration of East European Jews were confined to the East End of London, and while their numbers were so insignificant in relation to the rest of the British population,[63] Evans-Gordon chose to draw on obvious (medieval) anti-Semitic representations: 'Ten grains of arsenic in 1,000 loaves would be unnoticeable and perfectly harmless, but the same amount if put into one loaf would kill the whole family that partook of it.'[64] Similarly, in his 1903 book, *The Alien Immigrant*, he likened the 'influx' of immigrants to a plague of locusts.[65]

Even so, Evans-Gordon has been portrayed as a 'moderating influence' among some of the more 'unsavoury' anti-Semitic voices of the anti-alienist movement.[66] Committed to the anti-alien cause and the need to introduce immigration legislation, he insisted that the issue could not be one of overt anti-Semitism. Although, anti-Semitism was often at the foundation of the anti-alien debate, and was, I would argue, clearly a motivating factor for Evans-Gordon, expressions of overt anti-Semitism were not officially tolerated; indeed, the desire to quell an increase in anti-Semitism was an important factor in the decision to appoint a Royal Commission. Feldman argues that the Royal Commission on Alien Immigration was established in order to stem the growing agitation and anti-Semitism of the anti-alien movement roused by the BBL, LL and the popular East End press such as the *East*

London Observer.[67] Evans-Gordon was a central player in both in the Conservative Party and the BBL, acting as agitator and as conciliator. 'It was largely due to his efforts that a Royal Commission, of which he was a member was appointed to consider the alien question'.[68]

Finally giving in to repeated pressure from Evans-Gordon and Howard Vincent, Parliament agreed to an inquiry into the 'character and extent' of immigration. On 21 March 1902 the Royal Commission on Alien Immigration was appointed, and its task, while general, was to focus primarily on the 'character and extent' of immigration into London.[69] Henry James, Lord of Hereford (1828–1911), who had been Attorney-General in 1873–74 and 1892–95, was Chairman, while the other members included: Lord Rothschild, banker and philanthropist, regarded as 'the lay head of the [Anglo-Jewish] community';[70] Alfred Lyttleton, a lawyer and MP; Sir Kenelm Digby, an Under Secretary of State to the Home Office; Henry Norman MP; William Vallance, Clerk to the Guardians of Whitechapel; and Evans-Gordon.[71]

The examination of 175 witnesses began on 14 April 1902. Among these were nine Medical Officers of Health, the Chief Sanitary Inspector of Bethnal Green, two Vaccination Officers, a Customs Examining Officer, and physicians specialising in ophthalmic medicine. With the exception of Dr Hope, Medical Officer of Health for Liverpool, and James Niven, Medical Officer of Health for Manchester, all worked in London. Only one Port Medical Officer of Health was called to give evidence – Herbert Williams, of the Port of London.[72] This reflected the overwhelming focus of the Commission on overcrowding as the principal public health danger presented by immigrants. Generally the questions the medical witnesses were asked examined this issue, initially not focussing so much on medical and sanitary issues associated with immigrants, but on their opinions and observations of the current Registered Tenement Houses Bye-Law under the Public Health (London) Act 1891, and the laws which enabled sanitary authorities to deal with overcrowding. Via this line of enquiry the housing and sanitary conditions of both the newly arrived, 'green', and more established immigrants were extensively described, and their health and lifestyle illuminated in detail. 'Indigenous' infections which arose in overcrowded urban environments were part of these inquiries. Imported 'exotic' disease, or diseases such as trachoma which had been characterised as 'exotic' through association with migrants, was discussed very little by comparison.

However, even though a majority of the testimony related to the health and living conditions of immigrants once they had settled in London's East End, and to a lesser extent in Liverpool, Manchester and Glasgow, the Commission also responded directly to anti-alienists' concerns about their health on arrival and gathered evidence about the condition of immigrants at the ports. This was deemed necessary because of their 'impoverished and destitute condition', their general lack of sanitary 'habits', and, with American domestic and 'remote' medical inspections very much in mind, 'being subject to no medical examination on embarkation or arrival, are liable to introduce infectious diseases'.[73]

Yet, as only one Port Medical Officer of Health was questioned, with limited information solicited from the other medical professionals about health and disease at the ports, the introduction of infection through the ports cannot be seen as an overriding concern of the Commission. In addition, the evidence that was presented regarding the health of migrants on arrival and the occurrence of infectious disease amongst them revealed that although 'generally unclean', they did not present any great threat of infection. What was most evident in the testimony of the medical professionals involved with migrant arrivals was the notion that with increased capabilities, the Port Sanitary Authorities, in cooperation with local sanitary authorities, would be able to ensure that immigration posed no threat at all to the public health. All that was required, they argued, was more complete authority to detain vessels other than those suspected of carrying 'exotic' disease and to enforce a minimum standard of health and cleanliness in steerage accommodation.

One of the problems which most concerned the Commission was that when there was 'no suspicion or whisper of any epidemic or disease', Port Medical Officers did not board vessels or make any inspection of passengers or crew. [74] Medical Officers only boarded vessels which arrived from ports known to be infected with 'epidemic' disease, or when there was a positive reply to the question, 'Any sickness?' As there was a Port Medical Officer on duty twenty-four hours a day in London, who met the arrival of all vessels from on board the Customs launch, any case of sickness which was reported could be immediately attended to.[75] However, since the cessation of the General Cholera Order in 1895 there were no special powers relating to the inspection or observation of 'aliens'. Also since the abolition of the Quarantine Act, any special powers which the Port Sanitary Officer had obtained with regard to the enforced halting and detaining of vessels applied only to cases known or suspected to be cholera, yellow fever or plague. 'Exotic' disease remained distinctive from 'indigenous' infectious disease in the operation of port health, and retained with it particular jurisdiction. As Herbert Williams, the only representative of the Port Sanitary Authorities to testify, explained to the Commission:

> 7030. *(Chairman)* You board in order to find whether there are infectious diseases on board? – *(Williams)* We only board and inspect everyone on board when they come from places where there are exotic diseases.
> 7031. It is the question of exotic diseases and the class of diseases that come from specific ports; but it has nothing to do with alien immigrants? – No, not *per se.*[76]

Williams suggested that rather than extending inspections to monitor all immigrant ships, what was needed instead was increased authority to detain vessels with any serious infectious disease such as smallpox, scarlet fever, measles or diphtheria; in other words, broadening the powers which at that time only applied to 'exotic' diseases. He argued that although smallpox, for example, was an 'indigenous' disease, the last serious epidemic which occurred in England had, without doubt, been imported from Paris the previous June or July. 'That seems to me an example of how a disease existing in this country in a slight form might be added to or the effect increased by introduction from abroad'.[77] The categorisations of imported disease, then, were seen to have expanded beyond the 'traditional' binary, yet Williams did not comment on any additional category of disease imported by immigrants. His testimony revealed how port health practices continued to focus on the disease categories of 'exotic' and 'indigenous' as they had existed in the previous century rather than on categories of people or ships, migrants or merchants, for example.

Although the Port Sanitary Authorities now had jurisdiction over cholera, yellow fever and plague, they remained bound to remnants of the old system and continued to operate with one set of rules for one disease and one set for another. The power to order a vessel to 'come to', and most important to the Port Medical Officer of Health, the authority to detain a vessel at his own discretion, only applied to cases of 'exotic' disease. The powers of the Medical Officer were limited in cases of 'indigenous' disease, in comparison with those he possessed for diseases designated as 'exotic'. He could not detain a vessel on the mere suspicion of smallpox, for example; rather the ship's master, a layman, would have to report an illness first – a case of cold or lumbago often indicating the onset of an infection such as smallpox[78] – before an inspection could take place. The Medical Officer could not detain a vessel in order to inspect the passengers when no illness had been reported or the ship had sailed from a port which was not infected with an 'exotic' disease.

Williams emphasised that his role was to inspect vessels which arrived from infected ports or where cases of illness had been reported; beyond this he did not have the 'power to inspect with regards to individuals'[79] Thus, unless immigrants arrived on a vessel that fit either of the above two categories, Port Medical Officers of Health could and would not examine them. Even if they arrived in a 'filthy and unwholesome condition' covered with vermin, without specific cases of illness, there would be no inspection. Williams explained that vermin were neither particular to migrants – 'our soldiers in South Africa,'[80] for example, were infested with vermin – nor were lice an 'exotic' disease.[81] The responsibility of the Port Sanitary Authority was to prevent the importation of infectious diseases, not to ensure the general health and cleanliness of persons entering the port. The focus of port health was, in other words, still very much about particular diseases rather than particular people – the disease rather than the diseased. Williams suggested to the Commission that if it wished to improve the health of migrants who arrived into British ports, then the regulations relating to sanitation on board British vessels, legislated for under the Merchant Shipping Act, 1894, should be extended to foreign vessels destined for Britain. Since the cholera epidemic of 1892, the conditions on German and Dutch vessels had greatly improved. However the condition on board vessels from Libau, the main 'Russian' departure port,[82] remained 'abominable'. In 1902, according to Board of Trade statistics 34,918 aliens[83] arrived in Britain from 'Russian ports', which almost exclusively meant Libau.[84] Not only were the conditions highly unsanitary but, in order to maximise profits, migrants were crammed, for the duration of the three- to four-day journey, in the tightly overcrowded lower decks of the vessels. Williams illustrated this point with an example:

> On the 21st May [1902] the *SS. Hengest* [sic] of Aarhuus, from Libau, arrived at Gravesend with 171 Russian immigrants. The vessels left Libau on the 17th May. The immigrants were carried in the main

'tween decks ... an area of 2.3 square feet only per head being available... The quarters occupied by the immigrants were in a filthy condition, the floors being strewn with all kinds of refuse, and offensive liquid from the horses carried on the same deck had leaked through into these quarters. No attempt had been made at cleansing this space since the vessel had left Libau. Two temporary closets were provided, and both were used indiscriminately by the sexes. The only ventilation provided was by means of the bunker hatchways, and by two 12-inch ventilators, one of which was without a cowl, and closed.[85]

Such conditions, he argued, presented a greater threat to public health and increased the possibility of imported infectious disease. Williams recommended two solutions to the problem. Firstly, that a medical inspection of all persons on board ships bound for Britain should be undertaken at ports of departure, similar to the US procedure; and secondly, that the sanitary condition on board foreign vessels[86] should be brought under the standards of 'English' law.[87] In these ways the health risk of migrants arriving into British ports could be minimised.

So, the emphasis returned, after the crisis of 1892, to a focus on environment and place, focussing on 'infected' ports and shipboard sanitation, rather than on the bodies of people who disembarked in London and elsewhere. Williams's proposal implied an extension of the sanitary zone into the migrating localities of ships, seeing voyages, as Katherine Foxhall argues for an earlier period, as 'not simply a vector for disease' but potential 'productive physical and temporal space[s]'.[88] Thus, it was localities, and the places and people who connected them, that needed to be made to conform to sanitary norms and kept under sanitary surveillance. Immigrants, Williams argued, were only of interest where they entered into or linked these environments.

Yet in practical terms, as both the Chairman and Evans-Gordon pointed out, the conditions on board foreign vessels were outside the jurisdiction of the English System or British shipping regulations. 'Clearly our jurisdiction', Lord Hereford remarked, 'would come in as not allowing the reception of people, but that penalty would fall heavily on the immigrants. They would have to stop on board, or go back.'[89] Evans-Gordon, who had examined the American legislation, believed that legislation that focussed on immigrants and demanded carrier liability had greatly improved conditions on board vessels bound for the United States. He suggested therefore that the ability to refuse entry to Britain 'would have a further effect on the condition of the ship, because they would not bring them.'[90] Williams agreed that by prohibiting the landing of 'filthy aliens', the conditions on migrant vessels and therefore their condition on arrival would probably be improved. However, he pointed out that uncleanliness and vermin could easily be remedied by washing and disinfecting their bodies and clothes. Ultimately, he said, in his experience 'aliens' did not pose any particular or increased threat of infection,[91] particularly if medical and sanitary officers could be granted sufficient authority to regulate the environments migrants arrived at and proceed to.

Almost unanimously the medical witnesses who gave evidence to the Commission related that in their experience immigrants posed no more harm to the public health than the native population of the same class. In fact, although they often lived in overcrowded and unsanitary conditions – both on board migrant ships and in their dwellings once they had settled in Britain – immigrants generally displayed better results than the native population of the same class in population health indicators such as infant mortality, height and weight. What required reform, they repeated one after the other, was the authority of the sanitary authorities. Increase the power of the Medical Officers, they argued, and the perceived health problems presented by migrants would be satisfactorily addressed. They acknowledged that this could not solve the problem of overcrowding, but that was an issue that existed even without immigration. With few exceptions, the evidence provided by the London, Liverpool and Manchester Medical Officers and professionals stressed that the core concerns of the Commission relating to health were not specific to the 'alien' population but were 'really a question of surroundings – poverty, and so forth.'[92] Sanitary, not immigration, reform was what was required.

Perhaps the most strident advocate for this position was the most senior Medical Officer summoned to the Commission, Dr Shirley Murphy (1848–1923), the Medical Officer of Health for the Administrative County of London. He had been a member of the Royal Commission on Tuberculosis in 1901 and was the medical witness most extensively examined by the Alien Immigration Commission. Like all of his colleagues, he was thoroughly questioned about overcrowding and the sanitary conditions of immigrants in the East End of London as well as in the port; but he alone was asked the unusually direct question: did he believe that anyone should be refused entry on the grounds of poor health? Murphy rigidly maintained, despite a barrage of challenges from Henry Norman, that any person, regardless of nationality, should be treated equally. If an 'alien' arrived into the Port of London with any infectious disease – 'exotic' or 'indigenous' – Murphy argued that he ought to be taken to Denton and treated for the disease in the same way as an 'Englishman' would be treated; and once recovered he should be free to go, as would the 'Englishman'. He unequivocally opposed the refusal of entry upon medical grounds:

> 5011. *(Norman)* Do you, as the sanitary authority, see any reason, or not, for excluding on arrival a person whose physical condition would be such as to render him an undesirable member of the community? – *(Murphy)* If he is going to be a source of danger to the community, I should put him under restrictions on arriving here, that is to say, if the law would apply to similar people in this country – people suffering from the same malady.
>
> 5012. *(Norman)* What sort of disease would you put under these restrictions, which is not an exotic disease? – *(Murphy)* Smallpox and scarlet fever, for instance; people suffering from these diseases are not allowed to mix with other patients.[93]

Murphy reinforced the argument that the Port Sanitary System was fundamentally different from quarantine and American-style immigration controls, neither of which he believed had been particularly effective.[94] He emphasised that the same rational system of medical inspection, isolation of the infected and unobtrusive observation of the healthy by internal sanitary authorities was sufficient to provide a comprehensive barrier to the importation and spread of any infection without 'interfer[ing] with people's liberty' – regardless of their origin.[95] However, Norman and the Chairman, Henry James, remained unconvinced, and persisted in questioning Murphy about the differences in diseases brought by 'aliens'; asking if he would 'draw any distinction' between the diseases they carried from those of the 'ordinary foreign or English born subject arriving at our port'.[96] It was an important point, as the proposed restriction of immigration required the notion that the diseases of immigrants were essentially different from the diseases of the domestic population and required additional regulation and possibly separate supervision. Yet, Murphy remained firm, denying any difference for the purposes of disease prevention. He, like his fellow medical officers, was keen to ensure that all port health inspections remained under the control of the sanitary authorities, and argued that there was no reason why the 'exotic' immigrant could not be treated in the same way as the 'indigenous' population, just as sanitarians of the previous century had argued that 'exotic' disease could be prevented with the same stratagem as 'indigenous' disease.

However, as Port Sanitary Authorities did not have the same authority to act upon cases of 'indigenous' disease as they did in cases of 'exotic' disease, Evans-Gordon and other commissioners in favour of regulation argued that consequently 'indigenous' disease among 'filthy aliens' was capable of slipping through the defences. Norman and James suggested that the introduction of procedures similar to the American system of 'remote control' might reduce the number of 'diseased' aliens from arriving; but Murphy again stressed that proper sanitary conditions in the dwellings and neighbourhoods into which the migrants moved were the key to public health. Both Murphy and Williams argued for an extension of powers over 'indigenous' disease at the ports. In this way practices similar to those during the cholera epidemic could become the general practice. Any infection, such as measles, found present among a group of immigrants could then be isolated. The remaining passengers could be kept under observation at the discretion of the Port Sanitary Authorities, until they were released to the local sanitary authority of the district into which they moved.

Yet, even within this classification of 'indigenous', not all diseases were equal. The Royal Commission heard testimonies that argued for a hierarchy of these diseases. Smallpox, scarlet fever, measles, diphtheria and syphilis, for example, should be treated in the same way as any of the 'exotic' diseases, with complete authority granted to the port authorities to inspect and detain. Whooping cough, 'vermin', consumption (tuberculosis) and ophthalmia (trachoma) were examples of diseases that did not require additional powers of inspection as their 'native' sufferers were not subject to isolation.[97] These differences reflected both domestic regulations but also changing epidemiological patterns that saw diseases such as smallpox becoming much less common within the 'native' population and therefore more likely to occur when imported.

The most curious example included in the latter category was ophthalmia. Trachoma came to play a key role in the Commission's enquiries in relation to health and was the only disease singled out for special investigation. It was a highly contagious eye disease that has long formed part of the immigration narrative in the United States, becoming a central player in the 'immigrant experience' of the early twentieth century. The particular association between it and East European, mostly Jewish, immigrants in America has been well examined,[98] and its significance in the Royal Commission was directly related to the way it was perceived and treated in the United States.[99]

As discussed in the previous chapter, trachoma became central to immigrant screening procedures in the United States, as well as in informing popular perceptions of the 'contagious nature' of immigrants.[100] The disease affected only the health of the eye, but could cause blindness; it was, however, horribly unsightly and symbolised, in the very face of migrants, their 'diseased and contagious nature'. With the flick of an eyelid, it could be quickly diagnosed among the hundreds of immigrants who lined up for inspection after the arrival of a vessel, and it thus became synonymous with the arrival experience in America. Howard Markel remarked that the particular classification of trachoma as an immigrant disease led to the development of 'elaborate' international systems of inspection which controlled the movement of migrants across European frontiers.[101] These included the inspection of shiploads of migrants as they lined up at Britain's eastern ports before their departure for America.

The consequences of these American ways of thinking about trachoma, and the resulting inspections and deportations, created a deep impression on British anti-alien attitudes to the disease. These were clearly reflected in the Royal Commission on Alien Immigration where a number of witnesses were asked the same question – whether the 'alien' population was more subject to trachoma than the native population. Generally the reply was negative.[102] So great was the issue of trachoma that evidence was taken from two ophthalmic experts: William Lang, President of the Ophthalmological Society of the United Kingdom, and Francis Tyrrell, Surgical Officer to the Royal London Ophthalmic Hospital and Medical Officer to the London School Board. Tyrrell was summoned to give evidence; Lang volunteered to speak before the Commission with the specific purpose of refuting the testimony of Tyrrell. Called before the Commission in May 1902, Tyrrell claimed that trachoma was a disease particularly prevalent in the alien population and the restrictive laws which focussed on the disease in America had, along with the 'general uncleanliness' of the alien population, exacerbated the problem in London. Making his position clear, he told the Commission the story of when the Jewish Board of Guardians had sent him two young boys named Solomon and Elb who were suffering from trachoma. The boys arrived with a letter explaining that they had travelled to America from Russia, without transmigrating through Britain, but had been refused admission because of their disease. The letter asked if they could be treated and cured so that they might secure their entry into the United States. The boys represented a general trend, Tyrrell explained, that saw deported migrants who had travelled directly to America from the Continent locate to Britain for treatment. For this reason, he argued, cases of the disease among the native population had risen since the arrival of the aliens and that 'the Jewish people are peculiarly prone to trachoma.'[103]

Lang, incensed at learning what Tyrrell had said in this evidence, spoke to the Commission a year later, in May 1903. As one of the most senior ophthalmic surgeons in London, the boys and their letter, he explained, had in fact been sent to him. Tyrrell had been a junior outpatient surgical officer at the Royal London Ophthalmic Hospital (Moorfields) where the children were being treated and had been given the routine task of checking their progress on a daily basis by the more senior man. In addition to revealing his misleading evidence about the boys, Lang sought to object to all of Tyrrell's general statements about trachoma. It was, unlike Tyrrell had claimed, a curable disease and, Lang was keen to add, was 'not peculiar to Jews at all; it is universal all over the world.'[104] It was a disease more dependent on conditions than on race and 'the Jews, if they do bring it over, were not the originators of the disease; and they were not spreading it.'[105]

The Commission appeared to heed Lang's testimony. It, supported by the evidence of a majority of medical professionals who were examined, was reflected in the final report of the Commission which was submitted on 10 August 1903. The report clearly rejected the notion, as Tyrrell had laid out, that migrants had a particular role to play in the introduction or spread of trachoma, and noted its particular prevalence among 'poor children generally'. It stated that there was no evidence that the disease had been communicated from immigrants to the native poor, and that it was an indigenous infection that occurred as a 'consequence of the poor living resulting from poverty'.[106] Yet while the Commission had unmistakeably accepted the overwhelming evidence to this effect, it concluded, indulging its anti-alien members, that 'the desirability of permitting people suffering from this contagious disease into this country has to be considered'.[107]

This conclusion, along with the disease being the only one singled out specifically and repeatedly in discussion during the inquiry, clearly demonstrated that further meaning had been attached to the disease. With its obvious visibility, trachoma had come to symbolise the 'undesirable alien' in the United States, while in Britain it had come to symbolise a visible display of the fear that Britain was receiving migrants deemed unacceptable for entry to America. The disease represented the tight hold that anti-alienists perceived was connecting Britain's ports to American border controls. Although, as Williams had testified, under the present system smallpox among migrants was probably a greater public health threat,[108] trachoma had been imported from America as the symbolic manifestation of alien infection. It had become, as Markel remarked with regard to the United States, 'a powerful symbol of the threats of immigrant disease, dependency, and economic ruin against the body politic.[109] In this respect, it was almost entirely a *concept* of a disease which had been imported from the United States to Britain. It had become a symbol of Britain's reception of immigrants rejected from America on medical grounds and was an evocative image of 'undesirability' to be used by the anti-alien campaign.[110]

The acceptance of the idea that trachoma represented the diseased body of the migrant was subsequently extended onto a more generalised notion of the risk of diseased aliens. Although the Commission noted in its report that in relation to health 'we feel that we ought to place reliance upon the testimony of Dr Herbert Williams', particularly his statement that 'I cannot say that much infectious disease has come into the country among these people',[111] they recommended a focussed medical examination of immigrants at ports of arrival, and the deportation of those 'found to be suffering from infectious or loathsome disease, or mental incapacity' to their port of embarkation at the expense of the shipping company that had brought them.[112]

The intention was clear. Such regulations would have the ultimate effect not merely of excluding those deemed undesirable on medical grounds but would, in the first instance deter them, as in the United States, from attempting to enter and, most importantly, would act as a deterrent to shipping companies from carrying unhealthy passengers. They pushed the surveillance of migrant bodies outside and beyond the ports into a broader regulatory space distinct from the reaches of the sanitary zone. They also drew on standard public health models by seeking to reduce overcrowding and unsanitary conditions on board passenger vessels. Williams' concerns about the environment of steerage accommodation was recognised in the recommendation that called for further powers to regulate conditions on foreign immigrant passenger ships.[113]

Yet, the recommendation to legislate against entry on medical grounds did not coincide at all with the majority of medical testimony received by the Commission, and this did not go unnoticed by two members of the Commission, Kenelm Digby and Rothschild, who signed the report subject to memorandum. Digby's extended memorandum was seconded by Rothschild. He objected to 'some' of the recommendations made by the Commission which he believed did not align with either the evidence it received, or the conclusions which had been unanimously reached by the Commissioners. Central to these objections was the recommendation to restrict entry on health grounds:

> It has been proved in evidence as summarised in the Report, that there is very little illness amongst these immigrants, and that they are not found to have introduced any infectious or contagious disease. There is little or no evidence that lunatics come over with them, and the health of the immigrants after arrival here as proved by the Vital statistics given in evidence appears to be superior to that of the native population. No case therefore seems to have been made for any special measures for exclusion at the port of landing on the ground of health. Nevertheless, it seems desirable to have more definite and systematic inspection by sanitary officers, both of the ships in which the immigrants arrive, and of the immigrants themselves.[114]

Digby and Rothschild argued that the problem of alien immigration had proved to be essentially a local one and did not require solutions on a national level. Rather, it ought to be approached via existing public departments, without the need for the creation of a separate, national, Immigration Department. Rather than excluding immigrants, processes that would allow for their assimilation into a model of sanitary 'Englishness' would be more appropriate and proportional to the 'problem' they presented. A Jewish Board of Deputies Committee on the Alien Immigration Commission supported the unwillingness expressed by Digby and Rothschild to accept the recommendations. In their report they lamented that

> it would ... be most deplorable if the recommendation, made in the face of the mass of evidence to the contrary, serves to give colour to the popular impression that the diseased state of the immigrants of the past have necessitated the regulations mentioned.[115]

And yet, the recommendations were designed to do just that. The foundations of the anti-immigration platform, both before and throughout the Commission, were based on the leading allegation that immigrants were responsible for the housing, employment and poverty problems

in London's East End. Health, although not as central as social and economic factors, played an essential role in the debate, as much symboli-
cally as literally. It was a particularly important tool utilised by the BBL
and LL in the development of popular support for the immigration
debate, and one which easily tapped into traditional anti-Semitic paradigms, and it was no secret that any legislation resulting from the
Commission would be directed specifically at East European Jews. As
the Royal Commission published in its report, 'the excess is mainly
composed of Russians and Poles who belong for the most part to the
Jewish faith.'[116] The guiding force behind the particular Jewish focus of
the Commission's investigations and reports was Evans-Gordon, and it
was his particular political agenda which led to the inclusion of health
restrictions in the recommendations of the Commission.

Shortly after the Commission's findings were published and the
first Bill resulting from the enquiry was reviewed, the Secretary to the
Commission, F.E. Eddis, wrote a book based on his experiences and
observations during the Commission. Before sending the manuscript
for publication he forwarded a copy to the Home Office acknowledg-
ing his close involvement.[117] Their response was far from positive, stating that the book was 'quite intolerable' and 'objectionable' and that it
could only be supported for publication if approved by Rothschild,
Evans-Gordon and Lord Hereford. As a result, it was never published.
One reason it received such a hostile review was that it openly criticised the recommendations of the report and revealed what Eddis saw
as the biases within it:

> The Commission at the outset appointed one of their members to
> lead the attack against unrestricted immigration of foreigners. To
> Major Evans-Gordon, Member of the Parliamentary division of
> Stepney, was assigned this post of responsibility. All must admit that
> he brought to bear upon the issue an energy, an ability, and a dogged
> determination to do full justice to his side...[118]

This bias was noted by Rothschild, who according to Eddis had been
appointed to the Royal Commission as 'leader of the defence', and
who informed a deputation from the Jewish Board of Deputies that
'the general idea' of the Commission had always been to recommend
that a system similar to that which was in place in the United States
should be introduced in Britain.[119] Evans-Gordon, Rothschild insisted,
was heavily invested in the outcome of the Commission for his political career.[120] In other words, Evans-Gordon and the Conservative

Party had pledged to legislate on the issue since the previous century and the Conservative Prime Minister, A.J. Balfour, was equally committed to legislation by 1904–05. The decision to recommend the inclusion of medical restrictions in any immigration legislation was the result of the desire to replicate American legislation and also to honour the Conservative party pledge to legislate, championed primarily by Evans-Gordon. It was also, it seemed, a decision that had been made before and regardless of the evidence obtained by the Commission.

Aliens in the sanitary zone

Thus, after one failed Bill,[121] in which a number of clauses were not considered feasible,[122] a second Bill was introduced in 1905,[123] and the Aliens Act finally entered the statute books on 11 August 1905. In relation to health it stated that an immigrant would be considered 'undesirable' under the Act, if s/he [were] 'a lunatic or an idiot, or owing to any disease or infirmity appear[ed] likely to become a charge upon the rates or otherwise a detriment to the public'. It only applied to 'alien steerage passengers' and not to transmigrants in possession of 'prepaid through tickets'.[124] The composition of ports as acceptable spaces through which people could pass was thus defined. They were, as the legislation emphasised, not receptacles but conduits.

From the moment the recommendations of the Royal Commission were published, the Port Sanitary Authorities began to consider their position within the new system. Williams wrote in his monthly report to the Port Sanitary Committee in September 1903 that considering the work undertaken during the Cholera Order, responsibility for medical inspection under an Immigration Act should be given to the Port Medical Officers of Health. He stressed that these officers had particular and extensive experience of dealing with 'these immigrants' and that the 'machinery' within which they operated could be easily and immediately turned to the functions of the new legislation.[125]

As the second Bill presented to Parliament did not specify who the Medical Inspectors employed under the proposed Act would be, Williams and his provincial colleagues urged the government to amend the Bill so that all matters relating to the health of the ports would remain within their sole authority. They suggested an amendment to clause 2.(1) of the Bill, which proposed that the Secretary of State would appoint men with 'magisterial, business, or administrative experience' to posts within the new Immigration Department. Instead Williams and his colleagues suggested that the Medical Officers who had already carried out inspections at the ports were best suited for the job.[126] Although this clause was not amended in the Act, employment of the established Port Authorities was not precluded under it. The Act was passed in August 1905, but was not due to come into operation until 1 January 1906. In the intervening months the administrative and organisational structure of the Act had to be established, and the Port Sanitary Authorities were determined to maintain their dominion in the ports with a secure role in the new department.

Opportunely for the Port Sanitary Authorities, cholera yet again threatened to invade Western Europe at the end of summer 1905, apparently brought from the 'East' by Russian migrants. By September 'some cases' had occurred in Hamburg among 'Jewish emigrants'. The outbreak did not appear to be a 'serious one' but precautions were nonetheless put in place.[127] Again the Local Government Board issued regulations which permitted special authority, such as had been applied from 1892–95, with regard to 'risk' vessels, and instructed that Medical Officers detain vessels from certain 'infected' ports as well as 'all immigrants from other ports'.[128]

The verification of addresses was also re-introduced and the arrangement which had been entered into between the Poor Jews' Temporary Shelter and the Port of London Sanitary Authority was renewed. Throughout the 'crisis' period which lasted from September to late November (coincidentally the months between the passage of the Bill and the introduction of the Act), Medical Officers employed particular vigilance in boarding every vessel which arrived carrying immigrants. Not only was this deemed necessary as a public health precaution but it was also expected that additional checks would be needed for the increased number of 'undesirable types' of immigrants who would try to enter the country ahead of the implementation of the Aliens Act.[129]

The timing of the cholera outbreak was particularly advantageous to the Port Sanitary Authorities. The Local Government Board in London wrote to the Port Medical Officers of Hull, Grimsby and Tynemouth 'and also Dr. Leslie Mackenzie of Scotch LGB', reminding them to maintain a focus on migrants even if the risk of the cholera threat did not meet the usual level required for heightened defences.[130] At the same time, correspondences darted between the Port Sanitary Committee in London and the provincial Port Authorities, urging them to highlight their indispensable role and to place pressure on local Members of Parliament and other local authorities in order to ensure that Port Medical Officers became the designated Immigration Medical Inspectors.[131]

Keeping everyone in suspense, only one month before the Aliens Act came into force, the Secretary of State finally resolved who were to be appointed as Immigration Officers at the ports. The Immigration Officers responsible for all parts of the Act not referring to health, such as financial means and registration, were to be appointed from among the officers of the Customs Service. These duties were to be carried out in conjunction with their regular duties. As they ordinarily met every vessel which arrived at the ports, the role of Immigration Officer would be 'performed by Customs Officers as part of their normal duties'.[132]

In relation to health, while the suggested amendment had not been included in the legislation, the Secretary of State determined that medical inspection under the Aliens Act should remain within the existing structures of port health. The Aliens Committee, which was convened at the Home Office in order to prepare and implement the logistics of the Act, 'stated that they thought it not desirable that two bodies should be conducting a system of medical inspection'.[133] The Medical Inspector required at every immigration port would therefore be the Port Medical Officer of Health or, if there was none, the local Medical Officer of Health.[134] The potential to yet again have a system of dual authority at the ports was thus avoided and the Port Sanitary Authorities' dominion preserved.

Exactly what diseases the new Act was trying to exclude though was unclear from the start. In a memorandum to the Bill, Evans-Gordon questioned whether 'disease or other infirmity' referred only to chronic conditions or also 'meant to include persons suffering from infectious or contagious diseases'.[135] It was also not certain how the role of the new Immigration Medical Inspectors would intersect with the powers and duties already held by the Port Sanitary Authorities. An employee at the Office of Parliamentary Council advised that

> it will also be necessary to draw a distinction between infectious diseases and chronic diseases. The present policy of the Local Government Board, in accordance with treaties, is rather to enforce the landing of persons suffering from infectious diseases rather than to forbid it.[136]

These 'treaties' were the conventions signed at the International Sanitary Conferences of 1897 and 1903, in which Britain had again argued for the landing of healthy passengers from infected ships on condition they provided verifiable addresses and that infected individuals were isolated. Medical restriction to immigration did not strictly contravene these international conventions, nor did it interfere with international treaties regarding a state's right to repatriate foreign nationals. However, it did contradict the ideal of non-exclusion upon which Britain had constructed its arguments against quarantine since the 1850s.

The powers granted to the Port Sanitary Authorities in 1896 with regard to the treatment of vessels infected with 'indigenous' or 'exotic' diseases were not altered under the Aliens Act. The two categories of disease were not separated or distinguished in any way under the Act and the Port Medical Officers could deal with cases of either type of disease onboard an immigrant vessel without distinction. These vessels were therefore placed within an entirely separate category from non-immigrant vessels that could only be detained for inspection if there was a suspected case of 'exotic' disease. The geographical origin of disease therefore continued to be important but only in the case of increasingly rare cases of plague, yellow fever and, through special orders, cholera and only on non-immigrant vessels. Otherwise disease was identified as a threat only when it appeared within the bodies of immigrants. 'Indigenous' diseases such as tuberculosis, measles or typhus, for example, could pass through the ports in the bodies of sailors or traders without being monitored. It was the category of body which carried the disease, rather than the disease itself, which the new regulations sought to police.

To this effect, the practical duties of the Port Medical Officers of Health, as Immigration Medical Inspectors, were barely distinguished from their ordinary responsibilities. The only differences lay in the ships and people inspected and the scope of medical concern that could be exercised on immigrant arrivals.[137] The law remained the same regarding the way medical officers inspected non-immigrant vessels. The difference in inspection practices at the ports changed after the implementation of the Act only with regard to immigrant ships which were clearly defined as any vessel which carried 'more than twenty alien steerage passengers'. Immigration Medical Officers stopped and medically examined these vessels under the conditions of the Act, regardless of whether any illness was reported by the master or ship's surgeon. This definition of immigrant ships ensured that those vessels which were detained and examined under the special authority of the Aliens Act were specifically 'migrant vessels'. These vessels were legally defined in order to differentiate them from trading vessels which remained under the ordinary requirements of the Public Health Acts, and were detained and examined accordingly. Inspections were also focused only on 'alien steerage passengers' ensuring that no inconvenience was caused to passengers of a 'better class'. The unsanitary and threatening bodies of displaced poverty were thus resolutely separated from the orderly respectability of the first and second class passengers who continued to be allowed to move with ease within and through the lines that were being drawn around the nation. Thus, the English System – which had largely been developed to protect the commercial considerations of the ports – was maintained where trading vessels and individuals of economic standing were concerned. The contact zones through and between which they sailed could thus remain intact even as the national border tightened around the movement of poor migrants.

Even so, within the first year it was clearly evident that much of the medical evidence to the Royal Commission, as well as the predictions of Rothschild and Digby, had been well-founded; Evans-Gordon and his supporters on the Commission had drastically exaggerated both the scale of the immigrant health problem and the reduction in immigrant numbers that would be produced by medical restriction. In London, for example, only eighteen immigrants were deported for medical reasons in the first year of the Act, while a further twenty-two people who were considered medically 'undesirable' were later, on appeal, permitted to land.[138] The diseases or ailments which prohibited the landing of the eighteen unsuccessful immigrants, were not recorded. Trachoma, however, which had not previously been seen in Port Sanitary Authority monthly or annual reports, began to be mentioned with increasing frequency. Yet, as most evidence given to the Royal Commission had suggested, it failed to cause any notable problems as a disease imported by immigrants.

Thus, by the first decade of the twentieth century, the composition of Britain's ports and littoral had been reconfigured to accommodate both the conflicting demands of open fluidity – so long sought after – and a defined and policed border. The role of the Port Sanitary Authorities was key to its success. As well as their now established jurisdiction over imported 'exotic' disease, they had secured a place within the new immigration regulations and organisation, making them the sole medical authority operating within British ports. After over fifty years of opposition to policies of detention and exclusion at the ports, it was not any particular public health concern but the combination of a strong anti-alien campaign mounted largely by Conservative politicians and the impact of stringent American immigration laws which brought about the introduction of medical restrictions to immigration at British ports.

Notes

1 For further reading on the economic effect and reaction to immigration see Feldman, *Englishmen and Jews*; Garrard, *The English and Immigration*; Gartner, *The Jewish Immigrant in England*; Harris, 'Anti-Alienism, Health and Social Reform'; Holmes, *John Bull's Island*; Anne Kershen (ed.), *London: The Promised Land? The Migrant Experience in a Capital City* (Aldershot and Vermont: Avebury, 1997); Jan Lucassen and Leo Lucassen (eds), *Migration, Migration History, History: Old Paradigms and New Perspectives* (Berne: Peter Lang AG, European Academic Publishers, 1997); and Panayi, *Immigration, Ethnicity, and Racism in Britain.*

2 Memorandum from Marine Department of the Board of Trade, end April 1894, NA MT9/512/M7865.

3 Letter from Treasury Chambers to Board of Trade, 19 April 1894, NA MT9/512/H3435.

4 Public Health Act, 1896 [59 & 60 VICT.], 'An Act to Make Further Provision with Respect to Epidemic, Endemic, and Infectious Diseases, and to Repeal the Acts Relating to Quarantine'.

5 'Sanitary Report – Port of London Sanitary Committee with the Half-Yearly Report of the Medical Officer of Health for the Port of London, to 31st Dec, 1896,' *Port of London Sanitary Reports, 1896–1901*, p. 11, CLRO, 565B.

6 *Ibid.,* p. 12.

7 *Ibid.,* p. 13.

8 *Ibid.*

9 *Ibid.,* p. 14.

10 'Altogether there were recognised 36 cases of plague in Glasgow from the beginning of August to the end of September, 1900. Of these 16 proved fatal, a case mortality of 44.4 percent,' Bruce Low, 'Summary of the Progress and Diffusion of Plague in 1900,' *Thirtieth Annual Report of the LGB*, 1900-01 – *Supplement Containing the Report of the Medical Officer*, Appendix No. 18 (London: HMSO, 1902) [Cd. 747], p. 276.

11 'Memorandum on Precautionary Measures taken in 1899 to Prevent the Importation of Bubonic Plague into England and Wales..' *Twenty-Ninth Annual Report of the LGB*, 1899–1900 – *Supplement Containing the Report of the Medical Officer*, Appendix No. 15 (London: HMSO, 1901) [Cd. 299], p. 345.

12 *Sixth Annual Report of the Local Government Board for Scotland*, 1900, p. xxxvii.

13 Plague first became cause for concern in Britain when it appeared in Jeddah, Port Said and Alexandria in the first half of 1899. 'It was not, however, until August that the Board became at all disquieted about this disease.' In August official information 'was received' of the presence of plague in Porto, Portugal. *Twenty-Ninth Annual Report,* 1899–1900, p. xiv.

14 Theodore Thomson, 'Cholera and Alien Immigrants Arriving in the Port of London' (1905), NA MH19/237.

15 *Memoirs of Abraham Mundy – Secretary to the Jews' Temporary Shelter, 1897–1946,* vol. 1, chapter 1, pp. 1–2 (Jewish Museum, Finchley, Memoirs Box I); See also evidence of Stephen Moore, Chief Inspector of the Thames Police, *Minutes of Evidence – Select Committee on Emigration and Immigration (Foreigners)* (1889), 1841–6.

16 *Ibid.,* chapter 10, p. 1.

17 The Shelter was the principal immigrant aid organisation in London, through which, by 1903, 95% of the total number of Jewish immigrants arriving into London passed. Similar organisations operated in Hawich and Grimsby. See Evidence of Herman Landau, President of the PJTS, in *RCAI, Minutes of Evidence,* 16273.

18 General Committee Minutes, PJTS, 30 April 1893.

19 *Memoirs of Abraham Mundy,* vol. 1, chapter 13, pp 1–2; and *Jewish Immigrants,* Supplement to the PMOH Monthly Report, May 1894, CLRO, *PSCP* (March–May, 1894).

20 Evidence of Dr Herbert Williams, MOH Port of London, *RCAI, Minutes of Evidence,* 6189.

21 *Ibid.*

22 Letter from PJTS to the Town Clerk, Guildhall, 13 Feb. 1894, CLRO, *PSCP* (March–May 1894).

23 Williams, *RCAI, Minutes of Evidence,* 6189.

24 *Jewish Immigrants,* Supplement to the PMOH Monthly Report, May 1894, CLRO, *PSCP* (March–May 1894).

25 Executive Committee Minutes, PJTS, 18 June 1895.

26 Landau, *RCAI, Minutes of Evidence,* 16283.

27 For extended discussion of the economic impact of immigration in this period and its role in the rise of anti-alien sentiment see texts cited in note 2 of this chapter.

28 Tomas Haycraft, 'Alien Legislation and the Prerogative of the Crown', *Law Quarterly Review,* XIII (1897), 165–86, pp. 165 & 170.

29 Bill 55, 1898 [61 VICT.], 'A Bill to Regulate the Immigration of Aliens'.

30 *The Times,* May 24, 1898, p. 8a.

31 Aliens Registration Act, 1836 [6. WILL. IV].

32 *Report from the Select Committee on Emigration and Immigration (Foreigners)* (1889), p. xi.

33 Ports at which Aliens Lists were collected: Aberdeen, Belfast, Blyth, Bristol, Cardiff, Dover, Dublin, Folkestone, Glasgow, Goole, Grangemouth,

Granton, Greenock, Grimsby, Harwich, Hull, Kirkcaldy, Leith, Liverpool, London, Middlesbrough, Newcastle, Newhaven, Newport, North Sheilds, South Shields, Southampton, Sunderland, West Hartlepool. *RCAI, Appendix to Minutes of Evidence*, vol. III [Cd. 1741-I], Appendix IV.

34 Evidence of H.Llewellyn-Smith, Deputy Comptroller-General, Board of Trade, *RCAI, Minutes of Evidence*, 159.

35 In Llewellyn-Smith's evidence it was stated that an Officer of the Customs boards every vessel from Hamburg, Bremen, Rotterdam, and Libua – the major Continental migration ports for East Europeans. *Ibid.*, 146.

36 *Ibid.*, 155.

37 *Ibid.*, 167–8.

38 See Evans, Nicholas, 'Work in progress: Indirect passage from Europe Transmigration via the UK, 1836–1914,' *Journal for Maritime Research*, 3:1 (2001), 70–84.

39 *RCAI, Appendix*, TABLE V.

40 Llewellyn-Smith, *Minutes of Evidence, RCAI*, 122–30.

41 The precise date on which the arrangement was entered into is unclear.

42 Letter from PJTS to Board of Deputies, 8 Nov. 1898, LMA, ACC/3121/B02/01/003.

43 Landau, *RCAI, Minutes of Evidenc*, 16285.

44 Letter from the Board of Deputies to the Board of Trade, late 1898 (draft letter, undated), LMA, ACC/3121/B02/01/003.

45 Landau, *RCAI, Minutes of Evidence*, 16286.

46 *Ibid.* (16284–8 & 16410–14); and Letter, late 1898, LMA, ACC/3121/B02/01/003.

47 *Appendix to Minutes of Evidence, RCAI*, TABLES V & VII: *RCAI, Appendix*, TABLE VII titled, 'Statement of the number of aliens ascertained to have been *en route* to places out of the United Kingdom ... in addition to those described in the Aliens List'. The figures represented in both TABLES V & VII represent all migrants to all British ports. In TABLE V these figures are also broken down to represent London, Grimsby, Hull, Tyne Ports, Leith and Grangemouth, Newhaven and Dover. Similarly, the different nationalities of the migrants are broken down with regard to the number *not stated to be en route*. These are: Russians and Poles; Norwegians, Swedes and Danes; Germans; Dutch; French; Austrians and Hungarians; Italians; Roumanians; Other Nationalities.

48 Llewellyn-Smith, *Minutes of Evidence, RCAI*, 123.

49 As religion was not recorded at this stage one must assume that migrants from 'Russian and Poland' were, on the whole, Jewish refugees fleeing from the Pale of Settlement and the restrictive laws relating to Jews there.

50 Letter from the Board of Deputies to the Board of Trade, late 1898 (draft letter, undated), LMA, ACC/3121/B02/01/003.

51 *Ibid.*

52 See Hawkey, Customs Officer, *Minutes of Evidence, RCAI,* 1422–554.

53 Knepper, 'British Jews and the Racialisation', 61–79, p. 64.

54 Feldman, *Englishmen and Jews,* p. 91.

55 David Feldman, 'Jews and the British Empire, c. 1900,' *History Workshop Journal,* 63 (2007), 70–89, pp. 78–9.

56 *Ibid.*

57 Feldman, *Englishmen and Jews,* p. 288.

58 *The Times,* 1 Aug. 1901, p. 2f.

59 *The Times,* 30 Jan. 1902, p. 5e.

60 *Ibid.*

61 *Hansard, House of Commons Debates,* 29 Jan. 1902 [101], 1283.

62 *Ibid.*

63 'It may be argued that though the foreign population is large and increasing, it still remains small in proportion to the total population of London and insignificant in proportion to the population of the United Kingdom'. *Hansard,* 29 Jan. 1902 [101], 1274.

64 *Hansard,* 1274; Parallels may be drawn here with the 'blood libel' in which it was accused that the blood of murdered Christian children was used by Jews in the making of *matzah* (unleavened bread eaten at Passover).

65 William Eden Evans-Gordon, *The Alien Immigrant* (London: William Heinemann, 1903), p. 13.

66 Cecil Bloom, 'Arnold White and Sir William Evans-Gordon: Their Involvement in Immigration in Late Victorian and Edwardian Britain,' *Jewish Historical Studies: Transactions of the Jewish Historical Society of England,* 39 (2004), 155–63, p. 165.

67 Feldman, *Englishmen and Jews,* p. 288.

68 'Obituary Sir William Eden Evans-Gordon', *The Times,* 3 Nov. 1913, p. 11d.

69 *Report of the RCAI,* vol. I [Cd. 1741] p. v; also see *The Times,* 22 March 1902, p. 11f.

70 'Rothschild, Sir Nathan Meyer, 1840–1915', *DNB,* 1912–1921, p. 480.

71 F.E. Eddis was Secretary to the Commission.

72 Williams succeeded Collingridge as Medical Officer of Health for the Port of London in 1901, and held the post until 1916.

73 *Report of the RCAI,* p. 5 item 38.

74 Evidence of Thomas Hawkey, Examining Officer of Customs, London, *Minutes of Evidence, RCAI,* 1398.

75 *Ibid.,* 1387–403.

76 Williams, *Minutes of Evidence, RCAI,* 7030–1.

77 *Ibid.,* 6241.

78 *Ibid.,* 6092–3.

79 Chairman, *Ibid.,* 6130.

80 *Ibid.,* 6145.

81 *Ibid.*, 6165.

82 Libau was the Latvian port also known as Liepaja.

83 This figure represents both migrants *en route* and *not stated to be en route* in the Aliens List. *RCAI, Appendix*, TABLE VI.

84 See report of Evans-Gordon Report on visit to Eastern Europe, *Minutes of Evidence, RCAI*, 13349.

85 Williams, *Minutes of Evidence, RCAI*, 6176.

86 Migrants rarely, if ever, arrived into Britain from the Continent on British owned vessels. *Ibid.*, 6218.

87 *Ibid.*, 6208.

88 Katherine Foxhall, 'Fever, Immigration and Quarantine in New South Wales, 1837–1840,' *Social History of Medicine* (advanced access online, February 2011).

89 *Ibid.*, 6219.

90 *Ibid.*

91 *Ibid.*, 7131–42.

92 Evidence of Edward Hope, Medical Officer of Health for Liverpool, *Minutes of Evidence, RCAI*, 21466.

93 Evidence of Shirley Murphy, *Minutes of Evidence, RCAI*, 5011–2 & 5025.

94 *Ibid.*, 4917 & 5152.

95 *Ibid.*, 5005.

96 *Ibid.*, 5133, see also, 4992–5024.

97 Williams, *Minutes of Evidence, RCAI*, 6165 & 6239-41; and, Murphy, *Minutes of Evidence, RCAI*, 5013–5 & 5016–20.

98 Kraut, *Silent Travelers*; Kraut, 'Plagues and Prejudice, 65–90; Birn, 'Six Seconds Per Eyelid, 281–316; Markel, *Quarantine!*; Markel and Stern, 'All Quiet on the Third Coast, 178–82; Markel, '"The Eyes Have It"; Parascandola, 'Doctors at the Gate', 83–6; Solis-Cohen, 'The Exclusion of Aliens, 33–50.

99 Maglen, 'Importing Trachoma'.

100 See Birn, 'Six Seconds Per Eyelid'; and Markel, 'The Eyes Have It'.

101 *Ibid.*

102 See for example, Hope, *Minutes of Evidence, RCAI*, 21466; and Joseph Loane, Late Medical Officer of Health, Whitechapel, *Minutes of Evidence, RCAI*, 4706.

103 *Ibid.*, 3679.

104 Lang, *Minutes of Evidence, RCAI*, 20590.

105 *Ibid.*

106 *Report of the RCAI*, p. 11, item 71.

107 *Ibid.*

108 Williams, *Minutes of Evidence, RCAI*, 6239.

109 Markel, 'The Eyes Have it', p. 549.

110 Maglen, 'Importing Trachoma,' p. 96.

111 *Report of the RCAI*, p. 10, items 67–8.

112 *Ibid.*, p. 41, Recommendation, 4(g).
113 *Ibid.*, p. 42, Recommendation, 7.
114 *Ibid.*, 'Memorandum', p. 49.
115 ' Report of the Alien Immigration Committee of the London Committee of the Deputies of the British Jews on the Report of the Royal Commission on Alien Immigration', LMA, ACC/3121/B02/01/001.
116 *Report of the RCAI*, p. 40, item 262.
117 Letter to Home Office dated 2 May 1904, NA HO45/10241/B37811/15.
118 Proof, Eddis manuscript, NA HO45/10241/B37811/15B.
119 19 May 1904, NA HO45/10303/117267.
120 Arnold White Papers NMM WHI/166, Bedford Estate Office.
121 Bill 147, 1904 [4 EDW.7.].
122 Such as how was a 'person of notoriously bad character' to be determined and proved; see Holmes, *John Bull's Island*, p. 72.
123 Bill 187, 1905 [5 EDW.7.].
124 Aliens Act, 1905 [5 EDW.7].
125 CLRO, *PSCP* (Sept.–Dec., 1903).
126 Letter from the River Tyne Port Sanitary Authority to the Town Clerk, Guildhall, 21 June 1905, CLRO, *PSCP* (May–July, 1905).
127 CLRO, *PSCP* (Sept.–Dec., 1905).
128 19 Sept. 1905, CLRO, *PSCP* (Sept.–Dec., 1905).
129 *Ibid.*
130 See for example: Sept., 1905, NA MH19/237/104191/05.
131 Letter from the London Port Sanitary Authority to the Town Hall, Hull, 22 Aug. 1905, CLRO, *PSCP* (Sept.–Dec., 1905).
132 Letter from the Secretary of State to the Treasury, 9 Dec. 1905, NA HO162/1.
133 Draft memo, 'Aliens', CLRO, *PSCP* (Sept.–Dec., 1905).
134 NA HO162/1; see also Letter dated 9 Dec. 1905, CLRO, *PSCP* (Sept.–Dec., 1905).
135 Evans-Gordon, 'Memorandum on the Aliens Bill', 4 March 1905, NA HO45/117267/30.
136 Letter from the Office of Parliamentary Council to the Home Office, 13 March 1905, *Ibid.*
137 Draft memo, 'Aliens', CLRO, *PSCP* (Sept.–Dec., 1905).
138 Monthly Reports of the Port Medical Officer of Health for the Port of London, 1906, CLRO, *PSCP* (all file boxes 1906).

Conclusion

Yesterday marked World TB Day, the day in 1882 when Dr Robert Koch announced that he had discovered the cause of TB, the TB bacillus: 130 years later, London is the capital of TB in western Europe ... This is in part because of high immigration but also, according to the WHO's Dr Mario Raviglione, it is a result of the reluctance of the British government to comply with international standards and recommendations on notifications and the need for greater co-operation between departments, particularly the Department of Health and the UK Border Agency.[1]

The rise of tuberculosis and HIV infections in the last few years in Britain, appearing to be concentrated among immigrant populations, has elicited intense discussion about the advantages and disadvantages of introducing compulsory screening for these, and other, diseases as a requirement for entry into the country. Various Conservative politicians spent most of the first decade of the new millennium pushing for the introduction of pre-entry screening and succeeded in making it compulsory for migrants from a small number of countries who applied for visas of six months or longer to undergo TB testing before being issued a visa.[2] People arriving into Britain from all other countries or for periods of less than six months were not subject to compulsory screening but could be asked to undergo an x-ray for TB if they arrived at one of the two airports (Heathrow and Gatwick) equipped with the appropriate technology. While many believed this to be grossly inadequate, and pointed to numerous other countries, particularly Australia and the United States, as exemplars of successful medical inspection and exclusion legislation, others continued to support Britain's policies which focussed more on promoting public health initiatives, providing treatment under the National Health Service and allowing airport screening to remain voluntary. The exclusion of immigrants on grounds of health, argued those who opposed the introduction of more intensive screening at ports of arrival and departure, would not change the pattern of the epidemics. As an expert on HIV declared in an interview with the BBC in 2004, '[N]one of the countries that have introduced compulsory testing have halted their epidemics, and most have seen rapid increases'. [3] Rather, he and other critics of screening suggested that there ought to be a greater investment in existing public health programmes within Britain. [4]

Leading the rhetoric in current discussions about tuberculosis in Britain has been the idea that immigrants, or the 'non-UK-born', are predominantly responsible for the recent rise in incidents of the disease particularly in the capital. The concerns of the Home Office, expressed in a Ministerial Statement to the House of Commons in May 2012, emphasised how '[M]uch of the UK's TB burden is attributable to international migration. Around three quarters of TB cases in the UK occur in those born outside of the UK'.[5] This has been echoed in most of the mainstream media where the 'foreignness' of the disease has been underscored in all the lamentations and calls to action. Once acknowledged as a persistent scourge, a regrettable resident within the British population, the disease was thought to have been banished from the realm – no longer an indigenous disease, but something confined to 'exotic' locales far afield. There is simply no place for tuberculosis in twenty-first-century Britain's modern, clean and hygienic nation, these media reports (and the physicians they quote) insist. With their frequent descriptions of TB as 'Victorian' or 'Dickensian', they underscore the foreignness of the disease, signifying it as belonging to both a different time as well as a different place.[6] Indeed, the *Daily Telegraph* reported in 2010 that '"Victorian" living conditions among migrants are behind the rise'.[7] The question this prompts is whether the solutions to this once 'conquered' disease ought also to be 'Victorian', or whether the tools of 'modern' medicine dictate a different course. Unfortunately, public health and social reform are not quite as appealing as the image of 'a notorious killer in the Victorian era' and its defeat by medicine's magic bullets.[8]

However, the use of 'antibiotics and vaccinations', while certainly playing a role in current ways of thinking about prevention, are not central to the government's approach to the renewed threat of tuberculosis. Instead, the Home Office appears at this time to be reacting to the problem of 'imported' tuberculosis by increasing the system of

pre-entry TB screening for immigrants to a further sixty-six 'high inci-
dence' countries.[9] While this reorientation to off-shore medical inspection (which has not required any legislative changes) represents a
significant departure from previous practice, what is most striking
about current responses to imported infections is the *continuity* that it
reveals in both the flavour and the content of the recent debates with
those of a century ago. Tuberculosis has attracted the most media
attention over the past couple of years and, perhaps as a consequence,
has resulted in recent changes in screening procedures; yet there are
many other diseases that threaten to enter Britain from the 'outside'.[10]
Most notable are the potentially devastating 'emerging' infections such
as the recent and highly publicised dangers of SARS, 'Bird Flu' and
H1N1. The way all these diseases are being thought about, both in
terms of policy and practice as well as in public discourse, reveals a
similar set of problems to those that were tackled in the late nineteenth century. My intention here, however, is not to propose any wea-
risome and trite statement about history repeating itself, but rather to
suggest continuity – that the questions and problems that beset the
central actors and had their genesis in the period covered by this book
remain unresolved.

This study began with the assumption that in the late nineteenth
and early twentieth centuries, a 'medical panic' was focused at the
ports on the arrival of hundreds of thousands of immigrants and transmigrants. The inclusion of a clause in Britain's first immigration law,
the 1905 Aliens Act, which prohibited the entry of immigrants on
medical grounds, appeared to indicate, as it had in the United States, a
particular concern about the introduction into the native population
of a 'diseased' foreign population. Yet, by the time immigration restriction began to gain momentum in British politics in the years leading
up to the Act, the central platform adopted by anti-alien agitators was
not medical but economic, concerned with sweated labour, housing
and the undercutting of wages and prices. Unlike other countries
which received immigrants during this period of mass migration,
Britain did not respond to the arrival of thousands of aliens in the
unsanitary steerage holds of merchant steamships with the same
medical rhetoric of exclusion adopted with particular force in countries
such as the United States. The health condition of immigrants at the
moment of arrival, a powerful image in American anti-immigration
propaganda, did not, particularly after 1900, play a significant role in
the British anti-alien movement. However, the notion that immigrants

were the conductors of disease was not absent from Britain. Indeed, in the 1890s and into the twentieth century they were often considered to be the primary vector in the transmission of cholera and other infectious diseases. Yet, that immigrants posed a significant biological threat was never central to the rhetoric of anti-immigration or even public health.

Understanding why any potential medical threat posed by immigrants was not a significant part of the alien immigration debate at the turn of the twentieth century, yet still found its way into Britain's first immigration legislation, required instead an examination of nineteenth-century port health more generally. Britain maintained, particularly since the establishment of the Port Sanitary Authorities, confidence in a system of port health which opposed restrictive border controls such as quarantine. Any practices or rhetoric which were suggestive of exclusionary port health sat uncomfortably at the end of a half century of fervent anti-quarantinism. As such, this book has been an examination not only of the methods employed in Britain to prevent infectious diseases thought to be associated with immigration but, more fundamentally, of the development of an English System of prevention. This worked as an alternative to quarantine, sought to distinguish itself from Continental preventive practices, and allowed for a broader and more fluid 'sanitary zone' within which bodies and disease could move and yet be monitored and controlled. Within this framework, we have seen how conflicting ideas about sanitation and quarantine at the ports, as well as responses to immigration, were effectively questions about where the 'foreign' or 'exotic' dangers represented by cholera and, later, immigrants ought to be placed. Should they be kept outside and excluded, or could they be assimilated into the mainstream of domestic medical and sanitary practice alongside 'indigenous' infections and the 'native' population; and, ultimately, how would the control of these 'foreign' diseases and bodies shape or define the idea of an 'English sanitary zone'? Questions about how to categorise and control imported infections wrestled with how to identify amongst whom, with what and where lines of inclusion and exclusion should be drawn, and whether this was even possible with or around the nebulous notion of 'England' or 'Britain' within its broader global context at the turn of the twentieth century. There simply was no easy answer, nor was there any neatly drawn geographical line around the 'nation' which could help to define a biological 'us' and 'them'.

Current preparations and responses to disease threats grapple with these very same issues and questions as they extend into the twenty-first century. The medical screening of immigrants at Britain's international airports, as well as at the recently increased number of consular missions abroad, seek to place individuals and groups within categories of desirable and undesirable, as well as locate and describe the bounded territory into which they can or cannot enter. Depending on how a person, their health or origin is classified, medical inspection is either carried out relative to the Immigration Act 1971, particularly in the case of non-EEA migrants, or under other public health laws relating to ports.[11] Under both sets of laws medical inspections are primarily overseen by *local* authorities, who 'maintain a sanitary border ... defined by national and international law'.[12] Individuals are categorised using the results of x-ray or laboratory test results, and clinical diagnoses of Port Medical Inspectors, as well as geographical origin, defined either by birth or place of embarkation. As at the end of the nineteenth century, their disease is critical to how they proceed, or not, through the border. For instance, while long-term living conditions have been shown to be most important in the transmission and effects of tuberculosis, it, like trachoma at the turn of the twentieth century, has become intimately associated with immigrants, primarily Black African and South Asian.[13] The response by the authorities, therefore, has tended toward distancing and exclusion, as well as focusing on immigration or visa status, rather than looking at the environment in which many of the poorest immigrants live within Britain.

On the other hand, potentially pandemic imported emerging infections like SARS and H1N1 have not prompted prevention focussed specifically on immigrants; instead these diseases have come to fall within the category of 'national security' and 'biodefense' and are specifically named in the 2008 Cabinet Office *National Security Strategy* document. As a 'Tier One' National Security risk, a possible 'influenza-like pandemic' is categorised along with severe coastal flooding and other extreme weather and carries with it recommendations for the use and development of vaccines, international early warning systems and 'resilience' – something that '[T]he British people have repeatedly shown'.[14] Like other 'natural disasters' it does not carry an implication of blame which might attach it to a particular person or group. As such, airport screening relies on international information sharing focusing on sites and places of outbreaks and risk and the varied streams of people who flow through them. Quarantine is not recommended, and the *UK Influenza Pandemic Preparedness Strategy 2011* clearly states that

> there is no evidence of any public health benefit to be gained from meeting planes from affected countries or similar pro-active measures such as thermal scanning or other screening methods. Such measures are largely ineffective, impractical to implement and highly resource intensive.[15]

However, as a group of researchers from Loughborough University have pointed out in a number of recent articles, the growth of regional airports as connectors to global networks of travellers and other mobile populations has begun to change quite significantly the movement and patterns of disease. This explosion of traffic into and through regional airports has undermined both the way Britain's borders are defined and has also confused the reading of and ability to categorise the geographical origin of arriving passengers. With many regional airports being directly connected to major international hubs like Amsterdam, Paris and Frankfurt, with their extensive global network of destinations, 'the geographical complexities of individual journeys' is obfuscated and the categorisation of people by UK border controls is greatly complicated.[16] Heathrow and Gatwick, where most medical screening activity and technologies are still concentrated, continue to serve the largest number of international arrivals from all parts of the world. Yet the fact that regional airports were by 2008 receiving thirty-five per cent of all passengers – including forty-four per cent from the Western European EU, forty-seven per cent from Central America, thirty-six per cent from North Africa and twenty-six per cent from the 'Middle East' – has also not been reflected in disease preparedness at these airports where port health precautions have been downplayed, uncoordinated and even ineffective.[17] The Loughborough researchers argue that the enormous increase in air-passenger traffic to regional airports has forced a shift in the UK border that has 'effectively re-sited or "localise[d]" the border both across and within UK territory'.[18] They contend that because the control of infectious diseases remains focused on certain concepts of a 'sanitary border' that is primarily located at frontiers marked by major international airports or at 'offshore' screening facilities, the new 'border within' that is created by regional airports has been overlooked.

Their conclusions that the 'maintenance of a sanitary border involves a multiplicity of time-spaces that operate both within and beyond the territorial limits of a state', and the

> intrusive practices of screening and policing represent a return to the very exclusionary notions of 'inside' and 'outside' that the more liberalised regimes of cross-border mobility were designed to overcome

work just as well for the period covered by this book as they do for issues of disease prevention in present-day Britain.[19] This is because of the search for ways to conceive of 'internal' and 'external' spaces, of categories of 'desirable' and 'undesirable', and ways of understanding and dealing with dangerous infectious diseases that took root and have endured since the end of the nineteenth century. Port health is central to the conceptualisation of 'national' space and the 'imagined community' that lies within it.[20] While both of these remain unfixed and changing, Britain's response to imported infections continues to defy declarative controls like quarantine, and disease prevention continues to shift and maintain notions of what is 'inside' and 'outside' the border.

Notes

1 'Editorial – TUBERCULOSIS: Return of an Old Killer Needs a Concerted Global Response,' *The Observer (England)*, 25 March, 2012, p. 36.
2 The number rose from four in 2005 to eighteen at present (June 2012). They are: Bangladesh, Burkina Faso, Cambodia, Cote d'Ivoire, Democratic Republic of the Congo, Eritrea, Ghana, Kenya, Laos, Niger, Pakistan, Rwanda, Somalia, Sudan, Tanzania, Thailand, Togo, Uganda.
3 'Immigrants May Face HIV Tests,' *BBC News, World Edition*, Friday, 2 January 2004.
4 See for example: Evelyn Harvey, 'The No-Blame Game: TB Has Returned to London, But It Is Wrong to Blame Immigrants for the Capital's Public Health Crisis,' *The Guardian*, Monday, 28 January 2008.
5 *Ibid.*
6 See for example: Chris Smyth, 'A Dickensian Disease That Came Back from the Dead,' *The Times*, 3 June 2011; and Linsey Haywood, 'Why Biggest Killer in History Is Back,' *The Sun (England)*, 16 May 2012 (National Edition), p. 8.
7 Stephen Adams, 'London Is 'TB Capital of Europe,'' *The Daily Telegraph (London)*, 17 December 2010 (National Edition), p. 17.

8 Chris Smyth, 'Mass Jabs for Babies to Check TB Surge; Infection 'Out of Control' in Some Urban Areas,' *The Times*, 3 June 2011, p, 1,10.

9 These are: Afghanistan, Angola, Bhutan, Bolivia, Botswana, Burma, Burundi, Cameroon, Cape Verdi, Central African Rep, Chad, China (Including: Hong Kong SAR, and Macau), Congo, Djibouti, Ecuador, Equatorial Guinea, Ethiopia, Gabon, Gambia, Guinea, Guinea-Bissau, Guyana, Haiti, India, Indonesia, Ivory Coast, Kazakhstan, Kiribati, South Korea, Rep of Kyrgyzstan, Lesotho, Liberia, Madagascar, Malawi, Malaysia, Mali, Mauritania, Micronesia, Moldova, Mongolia, Morocco, Mozambique, Namibia, Nepal, Nigeria, Papua New Guinea, Peru, Philippines, Russian Fed, Rwanda, Sao Tome & Prince, Senegal, Sierra Leone, Solomon Islands, South Africa, Suriname, Swaziland, Tajikistan, Timorleste, Tuvalu, Uganda, Ukraine, Uzbekistan, Vietnam, Zambia, Zimbabwe.

   Danien Green (Minister of State (Immigration), Home Office; Ashford, Conservative), Written Ministerial Statement, 'Migrant Tuberculosis Screening,' *Hansard*, HC Deb, 21 May 2012, c47WS.

10 Alexander Caviedes, 'The Influence of the Media Upon Immigration Politics in the UK,' (2011). American Political Science Association 2011 Annual Meeting Paper. Available at Social Science Research Network: http://ssrn.com/abstract=1901809 (accessed 22 May 2012).

11 'The Public Health (Aircraft) Regulations 1979, the Public Health (Ships) Regulations 1979, and the Public Health (International Trains) Regulations 1994 are made under powers in the Public Health (Control of Disease) Act 1984 and are often referred to collectively as the port health regulations.' Health Protection Agency, *Health Activity Relating to People at Ports, Airports and International Train Stations in England* (2006), www.hpa.org.uk/webc/ HPAwebFile/HPAweb_C/1194947398177 (accessed 22 May 2012).

12 Lucy Budd, Morag Bell and Adam Warren, 'Maintaining the Sanitary Border: Air Transport Liberalisation and Health Security Practices at UK Regional Airports,' *Transactions of the Institute of British Geographers*, 36, 2 (2011), 268–279, p. 272.

13 Hiranthi Jayaweera, 'Health of Migrants in the UK: What Do We Know?' 15 March 2011, From the *Migration Observatory at the University of Oxford*, http://migrobs.vm.bytemark.co.uk/briefings/health-migrants-uk-what-do-we-know (accessed 25 May 2012).

14 Cabinet Office, *The National Security Strategy of the United Kingdom Security in an Interdependent World* (2008), Cm. 7291; See also, Laura K. Donohue, 'Biodefense and Constitutional Constraints,' *Georgetown Law Faculty Publications & Other Works*, Paper 677, http://scholarship.law. georgetown.edu/facpub/677 (accessed 25 May 2012).

15 Department of Health, *UK Influenza Pandemic Preparedness Strategy 2011*, www.dh.gov.uk/prod_consum_dh/groups/dh_digitalassets/documents/ digitalasset/dh_131040.pdf (accessed 25 May 2012).

16 Budd *et al.*, 'Maintaining the Sanitary Border,' p. 275.

17 *Ibid.*; and Adam Warren, Morag Bell and Lucy Budd, 'Model of Health? Distributed Preparedness and Multi-Agency Interventions Surrounding UK Regional Airports,' *Social Science and Medicine*, 74, 2 (2012), 220–227, pp. 226–7.

18 Budd *et al.*, 'Maintaining the Sanitary Border,' p. 273.

19 *Ibid.*

20 Benedict Anderson, *Imagined Communities: Reflections on the Origin and Spread of Nationalism* (London: Verso, 1983).

Bibliography

Archives and unpublished sources

London Metropolitan Archives

These records were held at the Corporation of London Records Office (CLRO) when research for this book was undertaken. They are cited throughout the book with their original CLRO reference code.

COMMITTEES: *Port of London Health Committee (Port Sanitary Authority before 1935)*

Minute Books	(1872–1935)[565 A–B].
Report Books	(1873–1934)[565 B].
Papers	(1872–1933)[608 D–F, 909 A].

Cholera Conference, 1893: Cholera Precautions for 1893 – Conference of Port Medical Officers of Health [MISC MSS/337/1–3].

Denton Hospital: Case Book (Infectious Diseases) 1884–1924 [6085].

General Orders re Medical Officer of Health and His Inspectors of Nuisances, 25 Sept, 1878 – Renewals of Powers, 1876–83 [MISC MSS/40.1].

'Hospital at Gravesend: Report to the Court of Common Council from the Port of London Sanitary Committee, 26 April 1883', *Printed Reports Index* [A/114F].

'Port of London Sanitary Committee – Return of Salaries and Other Expenses – 12 July 1894', *Printed Reports Index* [A/79F].

'Public Health Acts – Report of the Port of London Sanitary Committee – 15 May 1873', *Printed Reports Index* [A/113C].

Swann, W.G., *Port of London Health Authority, 1872–1972* (Guildhall: Corporation of London, 1972) [PD 108-2].

Glasgow City Archives – Mitchell Library

Customs and Excise:
CE60 Collector to the Board – Port Glasgow and Greenock.
Town Clerks Department:
DTC70/11/3 Reports of the Medical Officer of Health of the City of
Glasgow.

Jewish Museum, Finchley

*Memoirs of Abraham Mundy – Secretary to the Jews' Temporary Shelter,
1897–1946* [Memoirs Box I, 3 vols.].

London Metropolitan Archives

RECORDS OF THE ANGLO-JEWISH COMMUNITY:
Board of Deputies of British Jews [ACC/3121].
Jews' Temporary Shelter [LMA/4184].
(Minute and Letter Books also held by Professor Aubrey Newman,
University of Leicester)

National Archives and Records Administration (Washington, DC)

ARCHIVES I:
NARA s. exdoc. 58 (51-1), Congressional Serial Set, vol. 2685.
NARA s. exdoc. 52 (52-2), Congressional Serial Set, vol. 3056.
ARCHIVES II:
Consular Correspondence (Record Group 59):
Dispatches from Consuls, Glasgow, T207.
                          Liverpool, M141.
                          London, T168.

National Archives – Kew

Board of Trade
BT27   Commercial and Statistical Department and Successors:
Outward Passengers Lists.

Cabinet Office

CAB1   Miscellaneous Records.
CAB37   Photographic Copies of Cabinet papers.

Customs

CUST46   Board of Customs: Registered papers.
CUST49   Customs and Excise: Registered papers.

Foreign Office

FO83   Foreign and Commonwealth Papers and Predecessors: Political and Other Departments: General Correspondence.
FO93   Foreign Office and Foreign and Commonwealth Office: Protocols of Treaties.
FO146   Foreign Office: Embassy and Consulates, France: General Correspondence.
FO281   Foreign Office: Consulate, New York, United States of America: General Correspondence.

Home Office

HO45   Registered Papers (Sub-series: 1901–09).
HO144   Registered Papers, Supplementary.
HO162   Aliens Restriction Entry Books.

Ministry of Health

MH19   Local Government Board and Predecessors: Correspondence with Government Offices.
MH48   Local Government Board and Ministry of Health, Health Division: Public Health and Poor Law Service.
MH55   Health Division: Public Health Services: Registered Files and Other Records (Sub-series: Cholera).
MH113   Local Government Board and Predecessors and Successors – Medical Department: Official Memoranda and Senior Officers' Papers (Sub-series: 1871–1908).

Ministry of Transport

MT9   Marine Correspondence and Papers.
MT10   Board of Trade Harbour Department: Correspondence and Papers.

MT19   Admiralty Harbour Department: Correspondence and Papers.

MT23   Admiralty Transport Department: Correspondence and Papers.

Privy Council

PC1   Miscellaneous Unbound Papers, 1481–1946 (Sub-series: Public Health and Quarantine).

PC7   Letter Books.

PC8   Original Correspondence.

Royal College of Physicians, London

Letter: William Benjamin CARPENTER (1813–1885) to Benjamin Ward RICHARDSON – AUG 27, 1883.

Report and Notes of the Quarantine Committee, 1889 [2248/2–3].

Wellcome Institute for the History of Medicine

RAMC Collection: J. Fayrer, *Addresses and Papers, 1868–1888* [RAMC/ FAY].

Published official sources – pre-1914

Annual Report of the Supervising Surgeon-General of the U.S. Marine-Hospital Service, 1892 (Washington: Government Printing Office, 1893).

Copy of Dr. Theodore Thomson's Report to the Local Government Board on the Methods Adopted at Some Ports for Dealing with Alien Immigrants (London: HMSO, 1896) [137].

Correspondence Respecting the Sanitary Convention Signed at Dresden on 15 April 1893 (London: HMSO, 1893) [C. 7156].

Fifteenth Annual Report of the Local Government Board, 1885–6 – Supplement Containing Reports and Papers of Cholera Submitted by the Boards Medical Officer (London: Eyre and Spottiswoode, 1886) [C. 4873].

First Report of the Royal Sanitary Commission – With Minutes of Evidence up to 5 August 1869 (London: HMSO, 1870) [C. 281].

Fourteenth Annual Report of the Local Government Board, 1884–5 – Supplement Containing the Report of the Medical Officer (London: Eyre and Spottiswoode, 1885) [C. 4516].

Further Reports Respecting the Cholera Epidemic in Egypt and the Proceedings of the German Scientific Commission (London: Harrison and Sons, 1884) [C. 3996].

General Board of Health – Report on Quarantine, 1849, p. 137 [1070].

New York Chamber of Commerce – Report of the Special Committee of the Chamber of Commerce of the State of New York on Quarantine at the Port of New York During the Cholera of 1892 (New York: Press of the Chamber of Commerce, 1892).

Nineteenth Annual Report of the Local Government Board, 1889–90 – Supplement Containing the Report of the Medical Officer (London: HMSO, 1890) [C. 6141-I].

Proceedings of the International Sanitary Conference Provided for by Joint Resolution of the Senate and House of Representatives in the Early Part of 1881 (Washington: Government Printing Office, 1881).

Report from the Select Committee on Emigration and Immigration (Foreigners); Together with the Proceedings of the Committee, Minutes of Evidence, and Appendix (London: Henry Hansard and Son, 1889) [311].

Report of the Royal Commission on Alien Immigration (London: HMSO, 1903).
Vol. I – The Report [Cd. 1741].
Vol. II – Minutes of Evidence [Cd. 1742].
Vol. III. – Appendix to Minutes of Evidence [Cd. 1741-I].

Report of the Special Committee of the Chamber of Commerce of the State of New York on Quarantine at the Port of New York during the Cholera of 1892 (New York: New York Chamber of Commerce, 1892).

Report on the Mortality of Cholera in England, 1848–49 (London: HMSO, 1852).

Reports and Papers on the Port and Riparian Sanitary Survey of England and Wales, 1893–4; With an Introduction by the Medical Officer of the Local Government Board (London: HMSO, 1895) [C. 7812].

Reports on the Volume and Effects of Recent Immigration from Eastern Europe into the United Kingdom (London: HMSO, 1894) [C. 7406].

Reports to the Board of Trade on Alien Immigration (London: HMSO, 1893) [C. 7113].

Restriction and Prevention of Cholera (New Haven: Connecticut State Board of Health, 1890).

Return of Corporation Appointments (London: Charles Skipper & East Printers, 1879).

Second Annual Report of the Local Government Board, 1872–3 (London: Eyre and Spottiswoode, 1873) [C. 748].

Second Report of the Royal Sanitary Commission – Vol. I, The Report (London: HMSO, 1871) [C. 281].

Select Committee on Means of Improving and Maintaining Foreign Trade – Second Report (Quarantine) (1824) PP, VI. 165 [417].

Sixth Annual Report of the Local Government Board for Scotland, 1900 (Glasgow: HMSO, 1901) [Cd. 301].

Tenth Annual Report of the Local Government Board, 1880–81 – Supplement Containing Report and Papers Submitted by the Board's Medical Officer on the Use and Influence of Hospitals for Infectious Disease (London: Eyre and Spottiswoode, 1882) [C. 3290].

Thirtieth Annual Report of the Local Government Board, 1900–1 – Supplement Containing the Report of the Medical Officer (London: HMSO, 1902) [Cd. 747].

Twelfth-Annual Report of the Local Government Board, 1882–3 – Supplement Containing the Report of the Medical Officer (London: Eyre and Spottiswoode, 1883) [C. 3778-I].

Twenty-Nineth Annual Report of the Local Government Board, 1899–1900 – Supplement Containing the Report of the Medical Officer (London: HMSO, 1901) [Cd. 299].

Twenty-Second Annual Report of the Local Government Board, 1892–3 – Supplement Containing the Report of the Medical Officer (London: HMSO, 1894) [C. 7412].

Twenty-Sixth Annual Report of the Local Government Board, 1896–7 – Supplement Containing the Report of the Medical Officer (London: HMSO, 1897) [C. 8584].

Twenty-Third Annual Report of the Local Government Board, 1893–4 – Supplement Containing the Report of the Medical Officer (London: HMSO, 1894) [C. 7538].

Published official sources – post-2000

Cabinet Office, *The National Security Strategy of the United Kingdom Security in an Interdependent World* (2008), Cm. 7291, www.dh.gov.uk/prod_consum_dh/groups/dh_digitalassets/documents/digitalasset/dh_131040.pdf.

Danien Green (Minister of State (Immigration), Home Office; Ashford, Conservative), Written Ministerial Statement, 'Migrant Tuberculosis Screening', *Hansard*, HC Deb, 21 May 2012, c47WS.

Department of Health, *UK Influenza Pandemic Preparedness Strategy 2011*, www.dh.gov.uk/prod_consum_dh/groups/dh_digitalassets/documents/digitalasset/dh_131040.pdf.

Health Protection Agency, *Health Activity Relating to People at Ports, Airports and International Train Stations in England* (2006), www.hpa.org.uk/webc/HPAwebFile/HPAweb_C/1194947398177.

Journals and newspapers – pre-1914

The American Review
British Medical Journal (BMJ)

The Contemporary Review
Daily Mirror
Glasgow Medical Journal
Illustrated London News
The Lancet
Law Quarterly Review
Living Age
London Medical Gazette
Medical News (Philadelphia)
Medical Times and Gazette
National Board of Health Bulletin (Washington)
New York Medical Journal
The New York Times
The Nineteenth Century and After
North American Review
Practitioner: A Journal of Therapeutics and Public Health
Punch
Quarterly Journal of Microscopical Science
Sanitarian
The Times
Transactions of the Epidemiological Society of London

Newspapers and media sources – post-2000

BBC News, World Edition
The Daily Telegraph (London)
The Guardian
The Observer (England)
The Sun (England)
The Times

Published primary sources

Anon, 'Quarantine in Relation to Cholera', *The Practitioner – A Journal of Therapeutics and Public Health*, XI (1873), 222–9.
Anon, 'The Last Quarantine in England', *Living Age*, 6 (1897), 767–8.
Armstrong, S.T., 'Cholera at New York, and the New York Quarantine', *New York Medical Journal*, 56 (1892), 266–9.
Armstrong, S.T., 'Quarantine, and the Present Status of Quarantine Laws', *New York Medical Journal*, 56 (1892), 354–7.
Bartholow, Roberts, *Cholera: Its Causes, Symptoms, Pathology and Treatment* (Philadelphia: Lea Brothers & Co., 1893).

Bellew, H.W., *The History of Cholera in India from 1862–1881 – Being a Descriptive and Statistical Account of the Disease* (London: Trubner & Co., 1885).

Booth, Charles (ed.), *Labour and Life of the People – Vol. 1: East London* (London: Williams and Norgate, 1891).

Carroll, Alfred Ludlow, 'How Long Shall a Cholera-Infected Vessel Be Detained at Quarantine?', *New York Medical Journal*, 56 (1892), 350–1.

Chandler, W.E., 'Shall Immigration Be Suspended?', *North American Review*, 156 (1893), 1–8.

Chapman, John, *Cholera Curable: A Demonstration of the Causes, Non-Contagiousness, and Successful Treatment of the Disease* (London: J & A Churchill, 1885).

Collingridge, William, *The Duties of the Port Inspectors of Nuisances – For the Association of Public Sanitary Inspectors* (Whitechapel: Thos. Poulter & Sons, 1887).

Collingridge, William, 'Practical Points in the Hygiene of Ships and Quarantine', *Shipmasters Society, London*, 'Course of papers', no. 33, (London, 1894).

Collingridge, William, 'The Milroy Lectures – On Quarantine', *British Medical Journal*, Part 1 (13 March 1897), 646–9; Part 2 (20 March 1897), 711–14.

Cunningham, W., *Alien Immigrants to England* (London: Swan Sonnenschein & Co., 1897).

Death, James, *My Cholera Experiences* (Canterbury Street: The Sun Printing Company (Limited), 1892).

Doty, Alvah H., 'Quarantine Methods', *North American Review*, 165 (1897), 201–12.

Dyche, John A., 'The Jewish Workman', *The Contemporary Review*, LXXIII (1898), 35–50.

Evans-Gordon, Maj, William Eden, *The Alien Immigrant* (London: William Heinemann, 1903).

Fayrer, 'The Origin, Habits and Diffusion of Cholera, and What May Be Bone to Prevent or Arrest Its Progress, and Mitigate Its Ravages' *Addresses and Papers, 1868–1888* (1886).

Fayrer, Sir J., *The Natural History and Epidemiology of Cholera – Being the Annual Oration of the Medical Society of London, May 7, 1888* (London: J & A Churchill, 1888).

Gidney, Rev. W.T., *Alien (Jewish) Immigration* (London: London Society for Promoting Christianity amongst the Jews, 1905).

Girner, John H., Doty, Alvah H., and Drake, C.M., 'The National Government and the Public Health', *The North American Review*, 165, 493, (1897), 733–53.

Goodeve, E., 'On the International Sanitary Conference, and the Preservation of Europe from Cholera', *Transactions of the Epidemiological Society of London*, III (1866–67), 15–31.

Hamilton Fyfe, H., 'The Alien and the Empire', *The Nineteenth Century and After*, LIV (1903), 414–19.

Hansbrough, Henry C., 'Why Immigration Should Not Be Suspended', *North American Review*, 156 (1893), 220–7.

Harris, A. Wellesley, *A Detailed Report on the Precautions Adopted by the Southampton Port Sanitary Authority against the Importation of Cholera* (Southampton: 'Hampshire Independent' and 'Southern Echo' Offices, 1892).

Hughs, T.P., 'Sanitation vs Quarantine', *North American Review*, 155 (1892), 636–8.

Joseph Fayrer, *Recollections of My Life* (London: William Blackwood and Sons, 1900).

Klein, E., *The Bacteria in Asiatic Cholera* (London: Macmillan, 1889).

Klein, E. and Gibbes, H., *An Inquiry into the Etiology of Asiatic Cholera* (London, 1885).

Landa, M.J., *The Alien Problem and Its Remedy* (London: P.S. King & Sons, 1911).

Mackay, George A., *Practice of the Scottish Poor Law* (Edinburgh: W. Green & Sons, 1907).

Maclean, *Suggestions for the Prevention and Mitigation of Epidemic and Pestilential Diseases; Comprehending the Abolition of Quarantine and Lazarettos* (London, 1817).

MacNamara N.C. *Asiatic Cholera: History up to July 15, 1892 – Causes and Treatment* (London: Macmillan, 1892).

Mason, Patrick, *Tropical Diseases – A Manual of the Diseases of Warm Climates* (London: Cassell & Company, Limited, 1903).

Murphy, Shirley, *Infectious Disease and Its Prevention* (London: William Clowes & Sons Limited, 1884).

Notter, J. Lane, 'International Sanitary Conferences of the Victorian Era', *Transactions of the Epidemiological Society of London*, XVII (1898), 1–14.

Palmberg, Albert and Newsholme, Arthur, *A Treatise on Public Health and Its Applications in Different European Countries (England, France, Belgium, Germany, Austria, Sweden, and Finland)* (London: Swan Sonnenschein & Co., 1895).

Parkes, Louis C., *Infectious Diseases: Notification and Prevention* (London: H.K. Lewis, 1894).

Parkin, John, *Are Epidemics Contagious?* (London: Sampson Low, Marston, Searle, & Rivington, 1887).

Parsons, H. Franklin, 'Half a Century of Sanitary Progress, and Its Results', *Transactions of the Epidemiological Society of London*, xviii (1899), 1–38.

Powderly, T.V., 'Immigration's Menace to the National Health', *North American Review*, 175 (1902), 53–60.

Prudden, T. Mitchell, *The Story of Bacteria and Their Relations to Health and Disease* (New York: G.P. Putnam's Sons, 1889).

Sedgwick, William, *Principles of Sanitary Science and the Public Health with Special Reference to the Causation and Prevention of Infectious Disease* (New York: Macmillan, 1902).

Seeley, John, *The Expansion of England: Two Courses of Lectures* (London: Macmillan, 1914), First published in 1883.

Simon, John, *Public Health Reports*, vol. I (London: Offices of the Sanitary Institute, 1887).

Steiner, Edward A., *On the Trail of the Immigrant* (New York: Fleming H. Revell Company, 1906).

Steiner, Edward A., *The Immigrant Tide, Its Ebb and Flow* (New York: Fleming H. Revell Company, 1909).

Sykes, John F.J., *Public Health Problems* (London: Walter Scott, 1892).

'The Official Refutation of Dr. Robert Koch's Theory of Cholera and Commas', *Quarterly Journal of Microscopical Science*, 26 (1886), 303–16.

Thorne Thorne, Richard, 'On the Results of the International Sanitary Conference of Rome, 1885', *Transactions of the Epidemiological Society of London*, V (1886), 135–49.

Thorne Thorne, Richard, *On the Progress of Preventive Medicine during the Victorian Era* (London: Shaw and Sons, 1888).

Vought, Walter, *A Chapter on Cholera for Lay Readers – History, Symptoms, Prevention and Treatment of the Disease* (Philadelphia: The F.A. Davis Company, 1893).

Wall, A.J., *Asiatic Cholera: Its History, Pathology and Modern Treatment* (London: H.K. Lewis, 1893).

White, Arnold, 'A Typical Alien Immigrant', *The Contemporary Review*, LXXIII (1898), 241–50.

White, Arnold, 'The Jewish Question: How to Solve It', *North American Review*, 178 (1904), 10–24.

Whitelegge, Arthur, *Hygiene and Public Health* (London: Cassell & Company, Limited, 1893).

Willoughby, Edward F., *The Health Officer's Pocket-Book – A Guide to Sanitary Practice and Law for Medical Officers of Health and Sanitary Inspectors, Members of Sanitary Authorities, Etc.* (London: Crosby Lockwood and Son, 1893).

Wyman, Walter, 'Safeguards Against the Cholera', *North American Review*, 155 (1892), 483–91.

Published and unpublished secondary sources

Abbot, Edith, *Immigration – Select Documents and Case Records* (Chicago: University of Chicago Press, 1924).

Ackerknecht, Erwin H., 'Anticontagionism between 1821 and 1867', *Bulletin of the History of Medicine*, 22 (1948), 562–93.

Afkami, Amir Arsalan, 'Defending the Guarded Domain: Epidemics and the Emergence of an International Sanitary Policy in Iran', *Comparative Studies of South Asia, Africa and the Middle East*, 19, 1 (1999), 122–34.

Aldermann, Geoffrey, *London Jewry and London Politics 1889–1986* (London: Routledge, 1989).

Aldermann, Geoffrey and Holmes, Colin, *Outsiders and Outcasts – Essays in Honour of William J. Fishman* (London: Gerald Duckworth & Co., 1993).

Allen, Michelle, *Cleansing the City: Sanitary Geographies in Victorian London* (Athens: Ohio University Press, 2008).

Alroey, Gur, 'Out of the Shtetl. In the Footsteps of Eastern European Jewish Emigrants to America, 1900–1914', *Leidschrift*, 21–1 (2007), 92–122.

Anderson, Benedict, *Imagined Communities: Reflections on the Origin and Spread of Nationalism* (London: Verso, 1983).

Armstrong, David, 'Public Health Spaces and the Fabrication of Identity', *Sociology*, 27, 3 (1993), 393–410.

Arnold, David, 'Social Crisis and Epidemic Disease in the Famines of Nineteenth Century India', *Social History of Medicine*, 6 (1993), 385–404.

Atalic, Bruno, '1885 Cholera Controversy: Klein Versus Koch', *Medical Humanities*, 36, 1 (2010), 43–7.

Ayers, Gwendoline M., *England's First State Hospitals and the Metropolitan Asylums Board, 1867–1930* (London: Wellcome Institute of the History of Medicine, 1971).

Baldwin, Peter, *Contagion and the State in Europe, 1830–1930* (Cambridge: Cambridge University Press, 1999).

Bashford, Alison, 'At the Border: Contagion, Immigration, Nation', *Australian Historical Studies*, 120 (2002), 344–58.

Bashford, Alison, *Imperial Hygiene: A Critical History of Colonialism, Nationalism and Public Health* (Hampshire and New York: Palgrave Macmillan, 2004).

Bashford, Alison (ed.), *Medicine at the Border: Disease, Globalization and Security, 1850 to the Present* (London: Palgrave Macmillan, 2006).

Bashford, Alison and Gilchrist, Catie, 'The Colonial History of the 1905 Aliens Act', *The Journal of Imperial and Commonwealth History*, 40, 3 (2012), 409–37.

Bell, Duncan, *The Idea of Greater Britain: Empire and the Future of World Order, 1860–1900* (Princeton and Oxford: Princeton University Press, 2007).

Birn, Anne-Emanuelle, 'Six Seconds Per Eyelid: The Medical Inspection of Immigrants at Ellis Island, 1892–1914', *Dynamics*, 17 (1997), 281–316.

Bloom, Cecil, 'The Politics of Immigration, 1881–1905', *Jewish Historical Studies – Transactions of the Jewish Historical Society*, xxxiii (1995), 187–214.

Bloom, Cecil, 'Arnold White and Sir William Evans-Gordon: Their Involvement in Immigration in Late Victorian and Edwardian Britain', *Jewish Historical Studies: Transactions of the Jewish Historical Society of England*, 39 (2004), 155–63.

Booker, John, *Maritime Quarantine: The British Experience, c.1650–1900* (Hampshire: Ashgate, 2007).

Borneside, George H., 'Jaime Ferran and the Preventive Inoculation Against Cholera', *Bulletin of the History of Medicine*, 55 (1981), 516–32.

Brand, Jeanne L., *Doctors and the State: The British Medical Profession and Government Action in Public Health, 1870–1912* (Baltimore: Johns Hopkins University Press, 1965).

Brinkmann, Tobias, '"Travelling with Ballin": The Impact of American Immigration Policies on Jewish Transmigration within Central Europe, 1880–1914', *International Review of Social History*, 53 (2008), 459–84.

Brinkmann, Tobias, 'From Immigrants to Supranational Transmigrants and Refugees: Jewish Migrants in New York and Berlin before and after the Great War', *Comparative Studies of South Asia, Africa and the Middle East*, 30–1 (2010), 47–57.

Brocklehurst, Helen and Phillips, Robert (eds), *History, Nationhood and the Question of Britain* (London: Palgrave Macmillan, 2004).

Brockliss, Laurence and Eastwood, David (eds), *A Union of Multiple Identities: The British Isles, c.1750–c.1850* (Manchester: Manchester University Press, 1997).

Brown, Michael, 'From Foetid Air to Filth: The Cultural Transformation of British Epidemiological Thought, ca. 1780–1848', *Bulletin of the History of Medicine*, 82, 3 (2008), 515–44.

Budd, Lucy, Bell, Morag and Warren, Adam, 'Maintaining the Sanitary Border: Air Transport Liberalisation and Health Security Practices at UK Regional Airports', *Transactions of the Institute of British Geographers*, 36, 2 (2011), 268–79.

Bulloch, William, *The History of Bacteriology* (New York: Dover Publications, Inc., 1938).

Butterworth's Medical Dictionary (London: Butterworth's, 1978).

Bynum, W.F, 'Policing Hearts of Darkness: Aspects of the International Sanitary Conferences', *History and Philosophy of the Life Sciences*, 15 (1993), 421–34.

Bynum, W.F., *Science and the Practice of Medicine in the Nineteenth Century* (Cambridge: Cambridge University Press, 1994).

Bynum, W.F. and Porter, Roy (eds), *Companion Encyclopaedia of the History of Medicine* (London: Routledge, 1993).

Caviedes, Alexander, 'The Influence of the Media upon Immigration Politics in the UK' (2011). American Political Science Association 2011 Annual Meeting Paper. Available at Social Science Research Network: http://ssrn.com/abstract=1901809.

Chave, Sidney, *Recalling the Medical Officer of Health* (London: Hollen Street Press, 1987).

Coleman, William, 'Koch's Comma Bacillus: The First Year', *Bulletin of the History of Medicine*, 61 (1987), 315–42.

Coleman, William, *Yellow Fever in the North: The Methods of Early Epidemiology* (Madison: University of Wisconsin Press, 1987).

Colley, Linda, 'Britishness and Otherness: An Argument', *Journal of British Studies*, 31, 4 (1992), 309–29.

Collins, Kenneth, *Second City Jewry: The Jews of Glasgow in the Age of Expansion, 1790–1919* (Glasgow: Scottish Jewish Archives, 1990).

Concise Dictionary of Scientific Biography (New York: Charles Scribner's Sons, 1981).

Convery, Ian, Welshmand, John and Bashford, Alison, 'Where Is the Border?: Screening for Tuberculosis in the United Kingdom and Australia, 1950–2000', in Bashford, Alison (ed.), *Medicine at the Border: Disease, Globalization and Security, 1850 to the Present* (London: Palgrave Macmillan, 2006), 97–115.

Cook, Gordon C., *From the Greenwich Hulks to Old St Pancras: A History of Tropical Disease in London* (London: The Athlone Press, 1992).

Cook, Gordon C., *Disease in the Merchant Navy: A History of the Seamen's Hospital Society* (Oxford: Radcliffe Publishing, 2007).

Cooper, Frederick and Stoler, Ann Laura (eds), *Tensions of Empire: Colonial Cultures in a Bourgeois World* (Berkeley: University of California Press, 1997).

Cowen, Anne and Cowen, Roger, *Victorian Jews through British Eyes* (Oxford: Oxford University Press, 1986).

Crowther, M. Anne and White, Brenda, *On Soul and Conscience: The Medical Expert and Crime* (Aberdeen: Aberdeen University Press, 1988).

Cunningham, Andrew and Williams, Perry (eds), *The Laboratory Revolution in Medicine* (Cambridge: Cambridge University Press, 1992).

Currie, J.R. and Mearns, A.G., *Manual of Public Health – Hygiene* (Edinburgh: E & S Livingstone, 1945).

Curtin, Philip D., *Death by Migration: Europe's Encounter with the Tropical World in the Nineteenth Century* (Cambridge: Cambridge University Press, 1989).

Desmond, Adrian, *The Politics of Evolution: Morphology, Medicine, and Reform in Radical London* (Chicago: University of Chicago Press, 1989).

Donnan, Hastings and Wilson, Thomas M., *Borders: Frontiers of Identity, Nation and State* (Oxford and New York: Berg, 1999).

Donohue, Laura K., 'Biodefense and Constitutional Constraints', *Georgetown Law Faculty Publications & Other Works*, Paper 677, http://scholarship.law. georgetown.edu/facpub/677.

Doty, Roxanne Lynn, 'Immigration and National Identity: Constructing the Nation', *Review of International Studies*, 22, 3 (1996), 235–55.

Duffy, John, *The Sanitarians: A History of American Public Health* (Chicago: University of Illinois, 1990).

Dupree, Marguerite, 'Computerising Case Histories: Some Examples from the Nineteenth Century', *Medzin, Gesellschaft und Geschichte*, 11 (1992), 145–68.

Durey, Michael, *The Return of the Plague: British Society and the Cholera, 1831–2* (Dublin: Gill and Macmillam, 1979).

Dwork, Deborah, 'Health Conditions of Immigrant Jews on the Lower East Side of New York: 1880–1914', *Medical History*, 25 (1981), 1–40.

Ernst, Waltraud and Harris, Bernard, *Race, Science and Medicine, 1700–1960* (London: Routledge, 1999).

Evans, Nicholas. 'Work in Progress: Indirect Passage from Europe Transmigration via the UK, 1836–1914'. *Journal for Maritime Research*, 3:1 (2001), 70–84.

Evans, Nicholas J., *Aliens en Route: European Transmigration via the UK, 1836–1914'* (PhD thesis, University of Hull, 2006).

Evans, Richard, *Death in Hamburg – Society and Politics in the Cholera Years* (Oxford: Clarendon Press, 1987).

Fahrmeir, Andreas, Faron, Oliver and Weil, Patrick (eds), *Migration Control in the North Atlantic World: The Evolution of State Practices in Europe and the United States from the French Revolution to the Inter-War Period* (New York and London: Berghahn Books, 2003).

Fairchild, Amy, *Science at the Borders: Immigrant Medical Inspection and the Shaping of the Modern Industrial Labor Force* (Baltimore: Johns Hopkins University Press, 2003).

Farley, John, 'Parasites and the Germ Theory of Disease', in Rosenberg, Charles E. and Golden, Janet (eds), *Framing Disease – Studies in Cultural History* (New Jersey: Rutgers University Press, 1992), 33–49.

Farnie, D.A., *East and West of Suez – The Suez Canal in History, 1854–1956* (Oxford: Clarendon Press, 1969).

Fee, Elizabeth and Hammonds, Evelynn, 'Science, Politics, and the Art of Persuasion: Promoting the New Scientific Medicine in New York City', in Rosner, David (ed.), *Hives of Sickness – Public Health and Epidemics in New York City* (New Brunswick: Rutgers University Press, 1995), 155–96.

Fee, Elizabeth and Porter, Dorothy, 'Public Health, Preventive Medicine and Professionalisation: England and America in the Nineteenth Century', in Wear, Andrew (ed.), *Medicine in Society: Historical Essays* (Cambridge: Cambridge University Press, 1992), 249–75.

Feldman, David, *Englishmen and Jews: Social Relations and Political Culture 1840–1914* (Yale: Yale University Press, 1994).

Feldman, David, 'Was the Nineteenth Century a Golden Age for Immigrants? The Changing Articulation of National, Local and Voluntary Controls', in Fahrmeir, Andreas, Faron, Oliver and Weil, Patrick (eds), *Migration Control in the North Atlantic World: The Evolution of State Practices in Europe and the United States from the French Revolution to the Inter-War Period* (New York and London: Berghahn Books, 2003), 167–77.

Feldman, David, 'Jews and the British Empire, c. 1900', *History Workshop Journal*, 63 (2007), 70–89.

Feys, Torsten, 'The Visible Hand of Shipping Interests in American Migration Policies', *Tijdschrift voor Sociale en Economische Geschiedenis*, 7–1 (2010), 39–62.

Foxhall, Katherine, 'Fever, Immigration and Quarantine in New South Wales, 1837–1840', *Social History of Medicine* (advanced access online, February 2011).

Fraser, W. Hamish and Morris, R.J. (eds), *People and Society in Scotland – 1830–1914* (Edinburgh: Edinburgh University Press, 1990).

Garis, Roy L., *Immigration Restriction – A Study of the Opposition to and the Regulation of Immigration into the United States* (New York: Macmillan, 1927).

Garrard, John Adrian, *The English and Immigration 1880–1910* (London: Published for the Institute for Race Relations by Oxford University Press, 1971).

Gartner, Lloyd, *The Jewish Immigrant in England 1870–1914* (London: Allen and Unwin, 1960).

Gartner, Lloyd P., *American and British Jews in the Age of the Great Migration* (London and Portland, OR: Vallentine Mitchell, 2009).

Gilbert, Pamela K., *Mapping the Victorian Social Body* (Albany: State University of New York Press, 2004).

Gilbert, Pamela K., *Cholera and Nation: Doctoring the Social Body in Victorian England* (Albany: State University of New York Press, 2008).

Glover, David, *Literature, Immigration, and Diaspora in Fin-de-Siecle England: A Cultural History of the 1905 Aliens Act* (Cambridge: Cambridge University Press, 2012).

Goldberg, David and Rayner, John, *The Jewish People – Their History and Their Religion* (London: Penguin Books, 1987).

Goodman, Neville M., *International Health Organisations and Their Work* (Edinburgh: Churchill Livingstone, 1971).

Greenstein, Daniel, *A Historian's Guide to Computing* (Oxford: Oxford University Press, 1994).

Halliday, Stephen, 'Commentary: Dr John Sutherland, Vibrio Cholerae and "Predisposing Causes"', *International Journal of Epidemiology*, 31, 5 (2002), 912–14.

Hamlin, Christopher, 'Politics and Germ Theories in Victorian Britain: The Metropolitan Water Commission of 1867–9 and 1892–3', in MacLeod, Roy (ed.), *Government and Expertise – Specialists, Administrators and Professionals, 1860–1919* (Cambridge: Cambridge University Press, 1988), 110–27.

Hamlin, Christopher, *A Science of Impurity: Water Analysis in Nineteenth Century Britain* (Bristol: Adam Hilger, 1990).

Hamlin, Christopher, 'Predisposing Causes and Public Health in Early Nineteenth Century Medical Thought', *Society for the Social History of Medicine*, 5, 1, (1992), 43–70.

Hamlin, Christopher, 'State Medicine in Great Britain', in Porter, Dorothy (ed.), *The History of Public Health and the Modern State* (Amsterdam: Rodolfi, 1994), 132–64.

Hamlin, Christopher, 'Edwin Chadwick, 'Mutton Medicine' and the Fever Question', *Bulletin of the History of Medicine*, 70 (1996), 233–65.

Hamlin, Christopher, *Public Health and Social Justice in the Age of Chadwick: Britain, 1800–1854* (Cambridge: Cambridge University Press, 1998).

Hamlin, Christopher, 'Commentary: Ackerknecht and 'Anticontagionism': A Tale of Two Dichotomies', *International Journal of Epidemiology*, 38 (2009), 22–7.

Hardy, Anne, 'Public Health and the Expert: London Medical Officers of Health, 1856–1900', in MacLeod, Roy (ed.), *Government and Expertise – Specialists, Administrators and Professionals, 1860–1919* (Cambridge: Cambridge University Press, 1988), 128–42.

Hardy, Anne, 'Cholera, Quarantine and the English Preventative System, 1850–1895', *Medical History*, 37, 3 (1993), 250–69.

Hardy, Anne, *The Epidemic Streets: Infectious Disease and the Rise of Preventative Medicine* (Oxford: Clarendon Press, 1993).

Hardy, Anne, 'On the Cusp: Epidemiology and Bacteriology at the Local Government Board, 1890–1905', *Medical History*, 42 (1998), 328–46.

Harris, Bernard, 'Anti-Alienism, Health and Social Reform in Late Victorian and Edwardian Britain', *Patterns of Prejudice*, 31 (1997), 3–34.

Harrison, Mark, 'Quarantine, Pilgrimage, and Colonial Trade: India, 1866–1900', *Indian Economic and Social History Review*, 29 (1992), 117–44.

Harrison, Mark, *Public Health in British India: Anglo-Indian Preventative Medicine, 1859–1914* (Cambridge: Cambridge University Press, 1994).

Harrison, Mark, 'A Question of Locality: The Identity of Cholera in British India, 1860–1890', in Arnold, David (ed.), *Warm Climates and Western Medicine: The Emergence of Tropical Medicine, 1500–1900* (Amsterdam: Rodopi, 1996), 133–59.

Harrison, Mark, 'Disease, Diplomacy and International Commerce: The Origins of International Sanitary Regulation in the Nineteenth Century', *Journal of Global History*, 1, 2 (2006), 197–217.

Harvey, Charles and Press, Jon, *Databases in Historical Research – Theory, Methods and Applications* (London: Macmillan, 1996).

Higman, John, *Strangers in the Land: Patterns of American Nativism, 1860–1925* (New Brunswick: Rutgers University Press, 1988).

Hoerder, Dirk and Rössler, Horst, *Distant Magnets: Expectations and Realities in the Immigration Experience 1840–1930* (New York: Holmes & Meire Publishers, Inc., 1993).

Holmes, Colin, 'Joseph Banister's Anti-Semitism', *Patterns of Prejudice*, iv (1970), 29–32.

Holmes, Colin, *Anti-Semitism in British Society 1876–1939* (London: Edward Arnold, 1979).

Holmes, Colin, *John Bull's Island: Immigration and British Society 1871–1971* (London and Basingstoke: Macmillan, 1988).

Holmes, Colin (ed.), *Migration in European History* (Cheltenham: Elgar Reference Collection, 1996).

Holmes, Colin, 'Hostile Images of Immigrants and Refugees in Britain', in Lucassen, Jan and Lucassen, Leo (eds), *Migration, Migration History,*

History: Old Paradigms and New Perspectives (Berne: Peter Lang AG, European Academic Publishers, 1997).

Hope, E.W., *Health at the Gateway: Problems and International Obligations of a Seaport City* (Cambridge: Cambridge University Press, 1931).

Howard-Jones, N., 'Choleranomalies: The Unhistory of Medicine as Exemplified by Cholera', *Perspectives in Biology and Medicine*, 15, (1972), 422–33.

Howard-Jones, N., 'The Scientific Background of the International Sanitary Conferences, 1851–1938. 1', *WHO Chronicle*, 28 (1974), 159–71.

Howard-Jones, N., 'The Scientific Background of the International Sanitary Conferences, 1851–1938. 2', *WHO Chronicle*, 28 (1974), 229–47.

Howard-Jones, N., 'The Scientific Background of the International Sanitary Conferences, 1851–1938. 3', *WHO Chronicle*, 28 (1974), 369–84.

Howard-Jones, N., 'The Scientific Background of the International Sanitary Conferences, 1851–1938. 4', *WHO Chronicle*, 28 (1974), 414–26.

Howard-Jones, N., 'The Scientific Background of the International Sanitary Conferences, 1851–1938. 5', *WHO Chronicle*, 28 (1974), 455–70.

Huber, Valeska, 'The Unifaction of the Globe by Disease? The International Sanitary Conferences on Cholera, 1851–1894', *The Historical Journal*, 49, 2 (2006), 453–76.

Hutchinson, E.P., *Legislative History of American Immigration Policy 1798–1965* (Philadelphia: University of Pennsylvania Press, 1981).

Isaacs, Jeremy, 'D.D. Cunningham and the Aetiology of Cholera in British India, 1869–1897', *Medical History*, 42 (1998), 279–305.

Jacobson, Matthew Frye, *Whiteness of a Different Color: European Immigrants and the Alchemy of Race* (Cambridge: Harvard University Press, 1998).

Jayaweera, Hiranthi, 'Health of Migrants in the UK: What Do We Know?' 15 March 2011, From the *Migration Observatory at the University of Oxford*, http://migrobs.vm.bytemark.co.uk/briefings/health-migrants-uk-what-do-we-know.

Jones, Maldwyn, *Destination America* (London: Weidenfeld and Nicholson, 1976).

Kearney, Hugh, 'Four Nations History in Perspective', in Brocklehurst, Helen and Phillips, Robert (eds), *History, Nationhood and the Question of Britain* (London: Palgrave Macmillan, 2004), 10–19.

Kelly, Catherine, '"Not From the College, But through the Public and the Legislature": Charles Maclean and the Relocation of Medical Debate in the Early Nineteenth Century', *Bulletin of the History of Medicine*, 82, 3 (2008), 545–69.

Kershen, Anne (ed.), *London: The Promised Land? The Migrant Experience in a Capital City* (Avebury: Aldershot and Vermont, 1997).

Knepper, Paul, 'British Jews and the Racialisation of Crime in the Age of Empire', *British Journal of Criminology*, 47 (2007), 61–79.

Kraut, Alan M., 'Silent Travelers: Germs, Genes, and American Efficiency, 1890–1924', *Social Science History*, 12 (1988), 376–94.

Kraut, Alan M., *Silent Travelers: Germs, Genes, and the 'Immigrant Menace'* (Baltimore: The Johns Hopkins University Press, 1995).

Kraut, Alan M., 'Plagues and Prejudice: Nativism's Construction of Disease in Nineteenth- and Twentieth-Century New York City', in Rosner, David (ed.), *Hives of Sickness: Public Health and Epidemics in New York City* (New Brunswick: Rutgers University Press, 1995), 65–90.

Krista Maglen, *Investigating the Immigrant Experience: Poor Relief Applications, Computer Analysis and European Immigrants in Glasgow, 1881–1896* (MPhil Dissertation, Glasgow University, 1997–98).

Lattimore, Owen, *Studies in Frontier History: Collected Papers, 1928–1958* (Oxford: Oxford University Press, 1962).

Levitt, Ian, *Poverty and Welfare in Scotland 1890–1948* (Edinburgh: Edinburgh University Press, 1988).

Longmate, Norman, *King Cholera: The Biography of a Disease* (London: Hamish Hamilton, 1966).

Lowe, W.J., *The Irish in Mid-Victorian Lancashire: The Shaping of a Working Class Community* (New York: Peter Lang Publishing Inc., 1989).

Lucassen, Leo, *The Immigrant Threat: The Integration of Old and New Migrants in Western Europe Since 1850* (Chicago: University of Illinois Press, 2005).

Lunn, K. (ed.), *Hosts, Immigrants and Minorities: Historical Responses to Newcomers in British Society, 1870–1914* (Folkestone: Dawson, 1980).

MacLeod, Roy (ed.), *Government and Expertise – Specialists, Administrators and Professionals, 1860–1919* (Cambridge: Cambridge University Press, 1988).

MacLeod, Roy and Lewis, Milton, *Disease, Medicine and Empire – Perspectives on Western Medicine and the Experience of European Expansion* (London: Routledge, 1988).

Maglen, Krista, '"The First Line of Defense:" British Quarantine and the Port Sanitary Authorities in the Nineteenth Century', *Social History of Medicine*, 15 (2002), 413–28.

Maglen, Krista, 'A World Apart: Geography, Australian Quarantine, and the Mother Country', *Journal of the History of Medicine and Allied Sciences*, 60, 2 (2005), 196–217.

Maglen, Krista, 'Importing Trachoma: The Introduction into Britain of American Ideas of an 'Immigrant Disease', 1892–1906', *Immigrants and Minorities*, 25, 1 (March 2005), 80–99.

Markel, Howard, 'Cholera, Quarantines, and Immigration Restriction: The View from Johns Hopkins, 1892', *Bulletin of the History of Medicine*, 67 (1993), 691–5.

Markel, Howard, '"Knocking Out the Cholera": Cholera, Class, and Quarantines in New York City, 1892', *Bulletin of the History of Medicine*, 69 (1995), 420–57.

Markel, Howard, *Quarantine! East European Jewish Immigrants and the New York City Epidemics of 1892* (Baltimore and London: Johns Hopkins University Press, 1997).

Markel, Howard. "'The Eyes Have It": Trachoma, the Perception of Disease, the United States Public Health Service, and the American Jewish Immigration Experience, 1897–1924'. *Bulletin of the History of Medicine*, 74:3 (2000), 525–60.

Markel, Howard and Stern, Alexandra Minna, 'All Quiet on the Third Coast: Medical Inspections of Immigrants in Michigan', *Public Health Reports*, 114 (1999), 178–82.

Markel, Howard and Stern, Alexandra Minna, 'Which Face? Whose Nation? Immigration, Public Health, and the Construction of Disease at America's Ports and Borders, 1891–1928', *American Behavioral Scientist*, 42, 9 (1999), 1314–31.

Marks, Lara, 'Ethnicity, Religion and Health Care', *Social History of Medicine*, 4 (1991), 123–8.

Marks, Lara and Worboys, Michael, *Migrants, Minorities and Health – Historical and Contemporary Studies* (London: Routledge, 2000).

McDonald, J.C., 'The History of Quarantine in Britain in the Nineteenth Century', *Bulletin of the History of Medicine*, XXV (1951), 22–44.

McKeown, Adam, 'Global Migration, 1846–1940', *Journal of World History*, 15 (2004), 155–90.

Milne, Graeme J., 'Institutions, Localism and Seaborne Epidemics on Late-Nineteenth-Century Tyneside', *Northern History*, 46, 2 (2009), 261–76.

Morris, R.J., *Cholera, 1832: The Social Responses to an Epidemic* (London: Croom Helm, 1976).

Mullett, Charles F., 'A Century of English Quarantine, 1709 – 1825', *Bulletin of the History of Medicine*, 23 (1949), 527–45.

Newman, Aubrey (ed.), *The Jewish East End, 1840–1939* (London: Jewish Historical Society of England, 1981).

O'Driscoll, Patricia, "'Against Infection and the Hand of War…" The Early Years of the Port health Service', *Port of London: Magazine of the Port of London Authority*, 66 (1991), 65–9.

Ogawa, Mariko, 'Uneasy Bedfellows: Science and Politics in the Refutation of Koch's Bacterial Theory of Cholera', *Bulletin of the History of Medicine*, 74 (2000), 671–707.

Palmer, Sarah, 'Ports', in Daunton, Martin J. (ed.), *The Cambridge Urban History of Britain, Vol. III, 1840–1950* (Cambridge: Cambridge University Press, 2000), 133–50.

Panayi, Panikas, *Immigration, Ethnicity, and Racism in Britain 1815–1945* (Manchester: Manchester University Press, 1994).

Parascandola, John, 'Doctors at the Gate: PHS at Ellis Island', *Public Health Reports*, 113 (1998), 83–6.

Pelling, Margaret, *Cholera, Fever and English Medicine 1825–1865* (Oxford: Oxford University Press, 1978).

Pelling, Margaret, 'Contagion/Germ Theory/Specificity', in Bynum, W.F. and Porter, Roy (eds), *Companion Encyclopedia of the History of Medicine* (London: Routledge, 1993), 309–34.

Pickstone, John, *Medical Innovations in Historical Perspective* (Manchester: Macmillan, 1992).

Pickstone, John, 'Dearth, Dirt and Fever Epidemics: Rewriting the History of British 'Public Health', 1780–1850', in Ranger, Terence and Slack, Paul (eds), *Epidemics and Ideas: Essays on the Historical Perception of Pestilence* (Cambridge: Cambridge University press, 1992).

Pooley, Colin G, *Migration and Mobility in Britain Since the Eighteenth Century* (London: UCL Press Limited, 1998).

Porter, Dorothy, 'Public Health', in Bynum, W.F. and Porter, Roy (eds), *Companion Encyclopedia of the History of Medicine* (London: Routledge, 1993), 1231–61.

Porter, Dorothy, *The History of Public Health and the Modern State* (Amsterdam: Editions Rodopi B.V., 1994).

Robbins, Keith, 'The "British Space": World-Empire-Continent-Nation-Region-Locality: A Historiographical Problem', *History Compass*, 7, 1 (2009), 66–94.

Rose, Jonathan, *The Edwardian Temperament 1895–1919* (Ohio: Ohio University Press, 1986).

Rosen, George, *From Medical Police to Social Medicine: Essays on the History of Health Care* (New York: Science History Publications, 1974).

Rosen, George, *A History of Public Health* (Baltimore: MD, Johns Hopkins University Press, 1993).

Rosenberg, Charles E., 'Cholera in Nineteenth Century Europe: A Tool for Social and Economic Analysis', *Comparative Studies in Society and History*, VIII (1965), 452–63.

Rosenberg, Charles E., *The Cholera Years – The United States in 1832, 1849, and 1866*, With a New Foreword (Chicago: University of Chicago Press, 1987).

Rosenberg, Charles E., *Explaining Epidemics and Other Studies in the History of Medicine* (Cambridge: Cambridge University Press, 1992).

Rosenberg, Charles, 'Commentary: Epidemiology in Context', *International Journal of Epidemiology*, 38 (2009), 28–30.

Rosenberg, Charles E. and Golden, Janet (eds), *Framing Disease – Studies in Cultural History* (New Jersey: Rutgers University Press, 1999).

Rosner, David (ed.), *Hives of Sickness – Public Health and Epidemics in New York City* (New Brunswick: Rutgers University Press, 1995).

Rüger, Jan, 'Nation, Empire and Navy: Identity Politics in the United Kingdom, 1887–1914', *Past and Present*, 185 (2004), 159–87.

Rutland, Suzanne D., *Edge of the Diaspora – Two Centuries of Jewish Settlement in Australia* (Sydney: Brandl & Schlesinger, 1997).

Sanders, Ronald, *Shores of Refuge – A Hundred Years of Jewish Emigration* (New York: Schocken Books Inc., 1988).

Schepin, Oleg G. and Yermakov, Waldermar V., *International Quarantine* [Translated from the Russian by Boris Meerovich & Vladimir Bobrov] (Madison: International University Press, 1991).

Schonfield, Hugh J., *The Suez Canal* (London: Penguin, 1939).

Searle, G.R., *The Quest for National Efficiency – A Study of British Politics and Political Thought 1899–1914* (Oxford: Basil Blackwell, 1971).

Shah, Nayan, *Contagious Divides: Epidemics and Race in San Francisco's Chinatown* (Berkeley: University of California Press, 2001).

Shapiro, Leonard, 'The Russian Background of the Anglo-American Jewish Immigration', in Holmes, Colin (ed.), *Migration in European History* (Cheltenham: Elgar Reference Collection, 1996).

Solis-Cohen, Rosebud T., 'The Exclusion of Aliens from the United States for Physical Defects', *Bulletin of the History of Medicine*, 21 (1947), 33–50.

Stern, Alexandra Minna, 'Buildings, Boundaries, and Blood: Medicalization and Nation-Building on the U.S.-Mexico Border, 1910–1930', *The Hispanic American Historical Review*, 79, 1 (1999), 41–81.

Stoler, Ann Laura, 'Sexual Affronts and Racial Frontiers: European Ideas and the Cultural Politics of Exclusion in Colonial Southeast Asia', in Cooper, Frederick and Stoler, Ann Laura (eds), *Tensions of Empire: Colonial Cultures in a Bourgeois World* (Berkeley: University of California Press, 1997), 198–237.

Szreter, Simon, 'The Importance of Social Intervention in Britain's Mortality Decline c. 1850–1914: A Re-Interpretation of the Role of Public Health', *The Society for the Social History of Medicine*, 1, 1, (1988), 1–37.

Tomes, Nancy, *The Gospel of Germs: Men, Women, and the Microbe in American Life* (Cambridge: Harvard University Press, 1998).

Tomes, Nancy and Warner, J. H., 'Introduction to Special Issue on Rethinking the Reception of the Germ Theory of Disease: Comparative Perspectives', *Journal of the History of Medicine*, 52 (1997), 7–16.

Towner, Katrina, *A History of Port Health in Southampton, 1872 to 1919* (PhD thesis, University of Southampton, 2009).

Turner, Bryan S., 'Social Fluids: Metaphors and Meanings of Society', *Body and Society*, 9, 1 (2003), 1–10.

Wallis, Patrick and Nerlich, Brigitte, 'Disease Metaphors in New Epidemics: The UK Media Framing of the 2003 SARS Epidemic', *Social Science and Medicine*, 60, 11 (2005), 2629–39.

Warren, Adam, Bell, Morag and Budd, Lucy, 'Model of Health? Distributed Preparedness and Multi-Agency Interventions Surrounding UK Regional Airports', *Social Science and Medicine*, 74, 2 (2012), 220–7.

"Waterman", 'Guardians of the Port's Health. Part 1: The Defense against Communicable Disease', *The P.L.A. Monthly: Being the Magazine of the Port of London Authority*, 39 (1964), 402–5.

Watts, Sheldon, *Epidemics and History: Disease, Power and Imperialism* (New Haven: Yale University Press, 1997).

Watts, Sheldon, 'Cholera and the Maritime Environment of Great Britain, India and the Suez Canal: 1866–1883', *International Journal of Environmental Studies*, 63, 1 (2006), 19–38.

Watts, Sheldon, 'Cholera Politics in Britain in 1879: John Netten Radcliffe's Confidential Memo on "Quarantine in the Red Sea"', *The Journal of the Historical Society*, 7, 3 (2007), 291–411.

Weindling, Paul, 'A Virulent Strain: German Bacteriology as Scientific Racism, 1890–1920', in Ernst, Waltrand and Harris, Bernard (eds), *Race, Science and Medicine, 1700–1960* (London: Routledge, 1999), 218–34.

Weindling, Paul, *Epidemics and Genocide in Eastern Europe, 1890–1945* (Oxford: Oxford University Press, 2000).

Welshman, John, 'Compulsion, Localism, and Pragmatism: The Micro-Politics of Tuberculosis Screening in the United Kingdom, 1950–1965', *Social History of Medicine*, 19, 2 (2006), 295–312.

Wolstenholme, G and O'Connor, Maeve, *Ciba Foundation Report – Immigration: Medical and Social Aspects* (London: J & A Churchill, 1966).

Worboys, Michael, *Spreading Germs: Disease Theories and Medical Practice in Britain, 1865–1900* (Cambridge: Cambridge University Press, 2000).

World Health Organisation, *The First Ten Years of the World Health Organisation* (Geneva: World Health Organisation, Palais Des Nations, 1958).

Wright, Peter and Treacher, Andrew (eds), *The Problem of Medical Knowledge: Examining the Social Construction of Medicine* (Edinburgh: Edinburgh University Press, 1982).

Zolberg, Aristide, 'Matters of State: Theorizing Immigration Policy', in Hirschman, Charles, Kasinitz, Philip and De Wind, Josh (eds), *The Handbook of International Migration: The American Experience* (New York: Russell Sage, 2000), 71–93.

Zolberg, Aristede, 'The Archaeology of "Remote Control"', in Fahrmeir, Andreas, Faron, Olivier and Weil, Patrick (eds), *Migration Control in the North Atlantic World: The Evolution of State Practices in Europe and the United States from the French Revolution to the Inter-War Period* (New York: Berghahn Books, 2003), 195–222.

Zolberg, Aristede, *A Nation by Design: Immigration Policy in the Fashioning of America* (Cambridge MA: Harvard University Press, 2006).

Zylberman, Patrick, 'Civilizing the State: Borders, Weak States and International Health in Modern Europe', in Bashford, Alison (ed.), *Medicine at the Border: Disease, Globalization and Security, 1850 to the Present* (London: Palgrave Macmillan, 2006), 21–40.

Index

Note: 'n' after a page number indicates the number of a note on that page.